NURSING ADOLESCENTS

Other books of interest:

The Royal Marsden Hospital Manual of Clinical Nursing Procedures
A. P. Pritchard and J. Mallett
0 632 03387 8

Child Health Care: Concepts, Theory and Practice
B. Carter and A. Dearmun
0 632 03689 3

Playtherapy with Children: A Practitioner's Guide
S. Jennings
0 632 02442 9

Clinical Paediatric Dietetics
V. Shaw and M. Lawson
0 632 03683 4

Psychology of Pregnancy and Childbirth
L. Sherr
0 632 03388 6

Basic Child Psychiatry
P. Barker
0 632 03772 5

Child and Adolescent Psychiatry
M. Rutter, E. Taylor and L. Hersov
0 632 02822 X

NURSING ADOLESCENTS

Research and Psychological Perspectives

JAYNE TAYLOR

BSc, RGN, RHV, DipN, RNT
Head of School, Nursing and Midwifery, Suffolk College

DAVE MÜLLER

BEd, PhD, C. Psychol, FBPsS
Vice Principal, (Planning and Research) Suffolk College

**Blackwell
Science**

First published 1995

Set by DP Photosetting, Aylesbury, Bucks
Printed and bound in Great Britain by
Hartnolls Limited, Bodmin, Cornwall

DISTRIBUTORS
Marston Book Services Ltd
PO Box 87
Oxford OX2 0DT
(*Orders*: Tel: 01865 791155
  Fax: 01865 791927
  Telex: 837515)

North America
 Blackwell Science, Inc.
 238 Main Street
 Cambridge, MA 02142
 (*Orders*: Tel: 800 759-6102
   617 876-7000)

Australia
 Blackwell Science Pty Ltd
 54 University Street,
 Carlton, Victoria 3053
 (*Orders*: Tel: 03 347-5552)

A Catalogue record for this book is
available from the British Library

ISBN 0–632–03625–7

Library of Congress
Cataloging in Publication Data is available.

Contents

Preface

This important book brings together research and good practice in a much neglected field of health care. Insufficient attention is given to the needs of adolescents within the health care system, and in particular to the role of the nursing profession in offering specialized support. This reflects the difficulty that social scientists have had in defining the period of adolescence, and also the different legal frameworks within which the adolescent population exists.

The separation of nurse education and training into the four distinct branches, alongside developments in midwifery training, have not explicitly identified adolescents as a topic requiring specialized input. We would like to suggest that all four branches and midwifery would greatly benefit from an understanding of the needs of adolescents and the careful review of their health care needs. Within the field of developmental psychology the study of adolescents is a major area which has immediate practical relevance for all nurses and indeed midwives. It was this belief that led us to complete this book.

The two authors have used their knowledge and experience to bring together a psychological perspective on nursing adolescents. This is a particular strength of the book as there is considerable overlap between the methodology of psychology and the practical implementation of nursing care. The second theme which underlies the text is an emphasis on research and empirical methodology. The nursing profession now demands a research-orientated approach to nursing practice, and that texts which introduce subjects should themselves focus on research and be derived from and based upon it. Far from being an academic approach, the use of research highlights the overlap between researching findings and practice.

The first part of the book (Chapters 1 to 4) is concerned mainly with the nature and development of the adolescent individual. This section is relatively descriptive but brings together findings which are important in influencing nursing care.

Chapters 5 and 6 build upon this framework and provide practical support for the nurse in promoting health and in the provisions of adolescent health care. These two chapters highlight the need for much greater emphasis on research in this important area. Chapters 7, 8, 9 and 10 are more specialized and focus on major issues which relate specifically to adolescence. The information in these chapters is relevant to all branches of nursing and midwifery and has important implications for the provision of health care and for society in general.

The final chapter stresses the need for a much clearer commitment to developing research in this field, which is an exciting area for research and is to some extent relatively unexplored. The need for us to understand the health care requirements of adolescents and to provide for them is an important aspect of health care. It is through research, and the expertise and commitment of nurses and other health care professionals, that the longer term targets set by the government through the Health of the Nation initiative can be met. We hope that we have offered the reader enough background information to make the case for a greater understanding of adolescents and commitment to working with them.

Jayne Taylor
Dave Müller

Acknowledgements

To our families for continued support; to the publishers for their patience; and to Andy Smith and students of Suffolk College for photographic material.

Chapter 1
The Nature of Adolescence

We have given a great deal of thought about how to introduce this book which is about nursing, psychology and adolescence. We are aware, from our previous experiences of writing a similar book about children, that nurses are becoming more cognisant of the importance of psychological aspects of care. We are also familiar with the wealth of information available about the psychological development of adolescents. It is a process which has, after all, fascinated most of us either as we have lived through it, or when we think back on it. What we have found surprising, however, is that the application of psychological theory to the nursing care of adolescents has received very little attention. There is a paucity of nursing research and literature on the subject, and yet the special psychological needs of adolescents as a group, have been highlighted in many reports investigating the health services, over a number of years. Both the *Platt Report* (1959) and the *Court Report* (1976) acknowledged the need for adolescents to be considered as a discrete group of health care consumers, and more recently the Department of Health in its report *The Welfare of Children and Young People in Hospital* (1991) and the Audit Commission in *Children First* (1993) have reiterated this view.

We can only speculate about why as a group, adolescents have been largely ignored by the nursing profession. It is perhaps because adolescents do not usually comprise a separate group in terms of health care provision and there remains a tendency to view them either as older children or as young adults. Few doctors or nurses specialize in adolescent health care, although increasingly in psychiatry it is considered a speciality. Medical and nurse training programmes have tended to exacerbate the view that adolescents who require health care 'belong' to paediatrics or to a medical or surgical speciality depending on the nature of their illness and as a group they receive relatively little attention. In terms of hospital provision the decision about where they *do* belong appears to be more likely made on the basis of physical size, age and bed availability rather than to their psychological needs.

A second reason for the lack of information about nursing adolescents may be because adolescence is usually seen as a period of good health, and the numbers of adolescents who come into contact with therapeutic health services is small when compared to adults or younger children. It could therefore be argued that there are insufficient numbers to merit research or literature. We strongly dispute this view, both because of the interest that has been generated by this text, and because of evidence that suggests that in most general hospitals at any one time, there are sufficient numbers of adolescent patients to warrant specialist units where research could be undertaken (Burman 1985). We would suggest that there are not too few adolescents who come into contact with health services, but that they are so widely dispersed throughout hospital services that they are 'hidden'.

A third reason which is where we wish to begin our discussions relates to the very nature of adolescence itself. Defining what adolescence is and who adolescents are is problematic and controversial. There appears to be no general agreement about when adolescence starts, and even less about when it finishes. We can consider legal, physical, psychological and sociological definitions, but these provide limited and often contradictory opinions. Our starting point then is to consider the myriad of views about adolescence, with the aim of trying to begin to understand what most people agree is a complex period of the lifespan.

Definitions of adolescence

As we have already mentioned in our introduction to this chapter adolescence can be defined according to a number of criteria. We will for purposes of clarity discuss these criteria separately in order to give an overview of opinion. However we wish to start with one of the most comprehensive definitions given by Hauser *et al.* (1991) which states:

'The adolescent phase of the life cycle refers to a complex terrain of intersecting biological, intrapsychic, and social factors that together contribute to significant transformations in individual development.' (p177)

Whilst this definition does not tell us who adolescents are it does indicate that adolescence cannot be defined according to any one criterion, Hauser *et al.* (1991) go on to discuss how adolescents will follow a diversity of developmental paths under the influence of the factors they mention. It is useful, to consider that these development paths will lead to the achievement of a number of 'tasks' which we discuss in Chapter 4.

Hauser *et al.* (1991) also mention in their definition the word 'transformation', which is frequently used in relation to adolescence. Blair *et al.* (1962), for example, discuss the relative rates of transformation from childhood to adulthood in various cultures (a point we will discuss later on).

Other phrases which frequently appear in definitions of adolescence relate to the transitional nature of adolescence and to the maturation which takes places. The *Court Report* (1976) defined adolescence as 'the maturation of the child to the adult' and Jordan and Kelfer (1983) suggest that:

'it is an intense period of growth that represents the transition from childhood to adulthood.' (p149)

Rutter (1979) discusses this 'phase of transition from immaturity to maturity, from childhood to adulthood' and Blair *et al.* (1962), in a not altogether helpful definition, refer to adolescence as the 'period of transition' which 'begins at the end of childhood' and 'closes at the beginning of adulthood'! The United States Department of Health, Education, and Welfare (1979) provide an even more bizarre definition which focuses on transition:

'Adolescence is a transitional period between childhood and adulthood when the individual is no longer a child and not yet an adult.' (p1)

The problem with many of these views is that they do not provide those involved in policy decisions in health care with any definitive criteria for deciding who adolescents are. They tend to tell us who adolescents are not (i.e. children or adults) rather than who they actually are. They also suggest that adolescence has no value of its own, and that it is just a period of waiting. It could be argued that by suggestion they seek to reinforce the policies of many hospitals in the view that adolescence is not a distinctive period at all and is not therefore worthy of special consideration. We hope this is not the case, and in the next sections aim to clarify further criteria which may help to unravel this complex 'transformational', 'maturational', 'transitional' phase.

Chronological age

Adolescence can be defined according to chronological age. The World Health Organization (1977) states that adolescence begins at the age of 10 years and ends at 20 years. The starting point of adolescence has also been equated with the 'teenage' years (i.e. 13 years) or at some point between 10 and 13 years. Gesell *et al.* (1956), for example, suggested that the behavioural beginnings of adolescence begin at about 11 years.

The problems with defining this period according to age is that it suggests an abrupt starting and ending point. The idea that young people wake up on their tenth, eleventh or thirteenth birthdays and suddenly stop being children is somewhat mechanistic and does not account for the wide variations in psychological and physiological development. According to Kuykendall (1989) chronological age is not a viable option for defining adolescence because of the diversity in individual development. The *Court Report* (1976) also suggested that adolescence should be defined by development rather than age, and Gesell *et el.* (1956) discussed the notion that 'calendar time does not measure developmental time.' (p20)

Physiological development

Adolescence has also been defined according to physical criteria, with puberty taken as the starting point (Steinberg 1987; Windmill 1987; Buskist and Gerbing 1990). Hadfield (1962) also discusses puberty as 'the turning point between childhood and adult life'. However, taking puberty as a criterion does, as with chronological age, present certain problems: notably, that puberty can occur at any time between the ages of 9 and 16 years (Steinberg 1987). The *Court Report* (1976) reiterates this view, suggesting that between the ages of 10 and 15 years there are marked variations in development from pre-puberty to complete physical maturity.

There is also a marked difference in the age at which puberty occurs between girls and boys. Graham and Rutter (1985) suggest that menarche usually occurs at some time between the ages of 10 and 16 years in girls and testicular growth is usually complete between 13 and 17 years in boys. To take puberty as the beginning of adolescence would suggest that on the whole, girls reach adolescence before boys. However, physiological development does not necessarily correlate with psychological development: the idea that a 16-year-old boy, who may have left school but is not physically mature, is still a child, whereas a 10-year-old girl, by virtue of the fact that she has started menstruating, is an adolescent, is both controversial and inadequate in terms of planning services.

The end point of adolescence and the beginnings of adulthood in terms of physiological development is even more difficult to define, and is described by Buskist and Gerbing (1990) as 'fuzzy'. Steinberg (1987) suggests that adolescence ends physiologically with the completion and

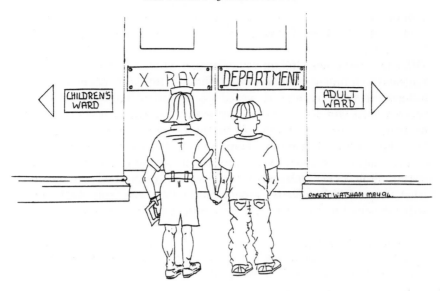

Fig. 1.1 Where does the adolescent fit in the hospital system?

ossification of the clavicle, which can occur between the ages of 18 and 25 years. This conjures up some rather bizarre pictures in terms of health care planning and the thought that the state of a clavicle could decide whether an individual receives care in an adolescent unit or an adult ward is clearly unrealistic!

Psychological development

In terms of using psychological development as a marking point for the beginning and end of adolescence, we are also faced with a number of difficult problems. Adolescence has become associated with the process of acquiring 'identity', a theme which we return to frequently throughout this book. Erikson (1965) believed that puberty and adolescence mark the beginning of a new stage of development which he described as *identity vs. role confusion*. During this stage, young people face identity crises, from which they will emerge with either a clear sense of identity or in a state of confusion about their future roles. The stage will eventually end in young adulthood, a stage which presents new challenges to the individual.

However, the view that adolescence ends when identity has been formed has been criticized by some. Marcia (1982) points out that although identity formation is distinctive during adolescence, it is not exclusive to it. He writes:

'If the termination of adolescence were to depend on . . . the formation
of an identity, then, for some, it would never end.' (p159)

There are also other difficulties in taking identity formation as a marker
for the development of health care policy. Identity formation is strongly
influenced by a number of variables, including parental–adolescent
relationships and socio-cultural pressures, and the process of identity
formation varies considerably from one individual to another. We discuss the work of Erikson and Marcia in more detail in Chapter 3.

A second major theory which relates to psychological development
during adolescence relates to cognitive changes which culminate in
what Piaget (1954) referred to as *formal operations*. This stage of cognitive development marks what Steinberg (1987) described as the

'ability to think logically, construct hypotheses, use ideas and imagi-
nation and distinguish from each other fantasies, ideas, beliefs,
probabilities and possibilities.' (p3)

The difficulty of taking formal operations as the starting point of adolescence is that not all individuals will reach this final and most complex
state of cognitive thought even during adulthood – it is not a universal
achievement (Overton *et al.* 1987). Some children at a relatively young
age will demonstrate formal operation thought, albeit in limited areas
(see Conger 1991). Clearly, Piaget's work could not be taken as the only
criterion for making health care policy in relation to young people,
although it certainly does appear to have some bearing on an individual's
ability to understand such things as concepts of illness and even death
(Swanwick 1990). We discuss the implications of Piaget's work in
Chapter 5.

Sociological criteria

Gunn (1970) suggests that adolescence is an artificially-created state
which has occurred because of the ever-increasing demands of a complex modern society. Certainly Gunn was not alone in the view that
young people require more knowledge of more things in order to be able
to cope with adult life. Hadfield (1962) also suggested that young people
require a greater knowledge in developed societies, and the process of
gaining independence therefore takes a longer period of time.

Rutter (1979) also discusses that it is society which determines the
nature, roles and expectations of adolescence, and that adolescence *per
se* is a socially created category. It is not however a universally accepted
category, and each culture and society will determine its own expecta-

tions of its youth. According to Rutter, adolescence as we currently know it is a product of the 'prevailing Western culture'.

The point made by Rutter does appear to have a great deal of relevance in any discussion about the nature of adolescence, as the universality of the stage is certainly doubtful. In some developing societies, for example, adolescence as a transitional phase between childhood and adulthood is non-existent, partially due to differing views of child and adult roles. In her account of family life in the third world Crehan (1992) suggests that the modern Western view of young people is not universal. In many parts of the world there is no clear distinction between the child's world and the adult world, particularly in terms of employment (typically an adult role in developed countries). Crehan points out that the idea of children selling their labour in the third world 'does not ... transgress accepted norms in the way that it does in the West' (p122).

Hadfield's view (1962) of the need for young people to go through a gradual process in order to gain independence can also be seen as a Western luxury. For example Hewitt (1992) gives a vivid account of the lives of abandoned children living on the streets of Brazilian cities, and illustrates how children are forced to become independent and undertake roles which are normally associated with adulthood. According to Ennew and Milne (in Hewitt 1992) one third of Latin America's 5 to 15-year-olds are economically active. Many turn to prostitution as a means of living. Not only are these children forced to work in order to live, they are also hunted down by the notorious 'death squads' who kill on average a child a day in Brazil.

In these circumstances, the idea of children taking their time to learn about adult life is alien, and does not reflect a true picture of life. It can be argued that for these, and many children throughout the world, there is no transitional period between childhood and adulthood where children can gradually learn to be independent from parents. Instead there is only the reality of independence and survival because there is simply no one on whom they can be dependent. This rapid introduction to the world of independence is not a new phenomenon. Blair *et al.* (1962) discussed the 'sudden transition' from childhood to adulthood in the third world which they suggested happens 'almost overnight'.

Perhaps we should not forget either that in Western societies our current view of adolescence as a transitional period is relatively new. In nineteenth-century Britain children as young as 7 years old were thrown into the world of adult responsibility by having to work for over 12 hours a day (Cox 1983). Rutter (1979) suggests that in these times adolescence meant something very different to its present meaning. Blair *et al.* (1962) argued that the period of adolescence was much shorter and lasted only a year or two. Young people married early and would take on adult family responsibilities when they were sometimes only 14 or 15 years old.

Finally we should remember that not all young people in Western societies today experience the comfortable transition between childhood dependence and adult independence. The growing number of homeless young people in Britain who are forced to earn money in whatever way they can means an early transition into the adult world of independence. Poverty can also limit opportunity for prolonging the transitional process of adolescence. Whilst education is now compulsory up to the age of 16 years, young people from lower socioeconomic classes are less likely to extend their formal education beyond that age (Giddens 1989). Additionally, uncontrollable variables can radically impinge on the period of adolescence and on a society's views and expectations of young people. War is one such variable, when a society may require young people to quickly assume adult roles. The diary of Zlato Filpovic (1994), a 13-year-old living in Sarajevo, is a vivid exemplar of this point.

Legal definitions

Legal definitions of adolescence are no more clear than any others that we have discussed in the preceding sections, in fact they are probably even more complex. We can find no legal definitions about when adolescence starts, and opinion about when a young person can assume adult roles is controversial, although young people under the age of 18 years are considered legally to be minors. It is, for example, possible to marry (with consent) at 16 years, and engage in heterosexual intercourse. It is not, however, legal to engage in homosexual intercourse until the age of 18 years. Nor is it possible to vote or purchase alcohol or drive a car, although it is legal to purchase cigarettes from the age of 16 years. These discrepancies clearly cause some confusion for young people.

Perhaps the most confounding issue which is of interest to all health professionals who work with adolescents is that of consenting to, or refusing, medical treatment. Under Section 8 of the Family Law Reform Act 1969, a minor aged 16 or 17 years can give consent to treatment (Dimond 1990). Subsequent events have deemed that children below the age of 16 years can also give consent 'at common law' under certain circumstances. The well known Gillick case, for example, has had a great deal of influence upon the issue of consent, as has the Children Act (DoH 1989), and we feel it is worth spending some time discussing these influences.

The Gillick case refers to the case of *Gillick v West Norfolk and Wisbech Health Authority* in 1985 when Mrs Gillick served notice on her local health authority forbidding any of their employees from giving contraceptive or abortion advice to any of her four daughters (then aged 5, 10, 12 and 13 years), whilst they were under 16 years of age, without her consent. The health authority refused to issue such instruction. What Mrs Gillick was attempting to do was to assert the absolute right of veto on the part of parents, in respect of her children under the ages of 16 years, to medical advice and treatment relating to contraception and abortion advice. After a well publicised legal battle, the courts decided that:

'as a matter of law the parental right to determine whether or not their minor child below the age of 16 will have medical treatment terminates if and when the child achieves a sufficient understanding and intelligence to enable him or her to understand fully what is proposed... Until the child achieves the capacity to consent, the parental right to make decisions continues...'
Lord Scarman (1985 All ER 402 at 423–424; 1986 AC 112 at 188–189)

Since the Gillick case several legal applications of the ruling have been made, and the concept of 'Gillick competence' has been argued. Of particular interest is that the original ruling in the Gillick case related to a competent minor *giving* consent to treatment and advice and not to *refusing* treatment.

In relation to giving consent the Children Act (DoH 1989) rules that:

'parental responsibility itself diminishes as the child acquires sufficient understanding to make his own decisions' (p9).

The situation, whilst not absolutely clear, does at least advise health care professionals that they should seek to determine whether minors are competent to make informed choices in relation to giving consent to examination and treatment, although Booth (1994) questions as to whether professionals will be prepared to engage in 'time-consuming investigations' of a child's ability to understand.

The issue of whether minors in law can refuse treatment is however much more complex and was brought to light in another well publicised case (*Re W*) involving a 16-year-old girl with anorexia nervosa who was refusing treatment (see Huchesson 1992). The ruling in this case was that there is a difference in terms of consenting and refusing and, whilst reiterating that a minor who is Gillick competent has the right to consent to treatment and that consent cannot be overridden by parents (although it can be overridden by the court), the court ruled that no minor 'of whatever age' has an absolute right to make decisions on medical treatment, especially when that decision is refusal (see Shield and Baum 1994).

The ruling relating to refusal of treatment clearly raises some important questions in relation to adolescents undertaking (or not) adult roles and responsibilities, and adds to the confusing legal parameters as to what adolescents can and cannot do. Although the court did emphasize that those with parental responsibility and the courts should consider carefully the wishes of the minor before overriding refusal, we are left with the situation that a minor under 16 years who is 'Gillick competent' can consent to major, life-threatening therapy, even if parents do not consent, whereas a minor under 18 years does not have legal abilities to refuse the same treatment if parents (with the backing of the court) deem that such treatment should be carried out.

It is perhaps worth mentioning that there are specific provisions under the Mental Health Act 1983 which relate to minors under the age of 16 years, as well as provisions under the Children Act 1989 relating specifically to psychiatric and medical treatment (see The Children Act, Schedule 3, paragraph 5).

Opinion about adolescence

During the following chapters we highlight some of the problems which occur during adolescence. Some of these problems, for example the eating disorders, peak during this period. Others, such as substance abuse, are thought to start during the adolescent years. These problems, and others such as antisocial behaviour, mark out adolescence as being a period of conflict, or as a time of 'storm and stress'. This latter term was favoured by Hall in 1904; he saw adolescence as being characterized by instability, turmoil and disturbance.

The view of adolescence as a time of conflict has been favoured for a number of years. Eppel and Eppel (1966) in their discussion of images of adolescence over time suggested that even before adolescents became 'a major target for commercial exploitation' (p3) during the 1930s, adults had been concerned about the 'declining morals of the younger generation'. Anna Freud (1958) held a similar view of adolescence as being a period of extreme turmoil, the manifestations of which she likened to the 'symptom formation of the neurotic, psychotic or dissocial order'. Likening the manifestations of adolescence to mental disorder was in fact a popular image at the time, until Erikson (1965) suggested that what may appear to be neurosis was in reality a crisis which would tend to resolve, and which may be constructive in contributing towards the process of identity formation.

The positive side of adolescence was seen by only a minority of authors during the 1950s and 1960s, with most opinions favouring the negative image of youth and, in particular, declining morality. In 1959 for example, the British Medical Association made adolescence their subject of the year and, whilst acknowledging that the vast majority of youth were on the whole 'cheerful, tolerant, sensible [and] non-delinquent', the focus of their report published in 1961, was of the adolescent who has 'learned no definite moral standards from his parents, is contemptuous of the law, easily bored and wants no more in the way of a career than a job of which the material benefits are more important than its power to satisfy' (BMA 1961). The decline of moral standards was also the theme chosen by Mr Butler, then the Home Secretary, in his opening address to the National Union of Teachers conference in 1960 (see Eppel and Eppel 1966). He spoke of the trouble of a 'moral character among our young people', and placed the blame for declining moral standards firmly at the door of the enhanced opportunity afforded to adolescents. Prosperity according to Butler brought with it its own 'evils'. Certainly the pejorative view of the time was one that deplored what was seen as the deterioration of adolescent morality.

The negative view of adolescence was probably reinforced even more during the 1960s and 1970s with the 'flower power' era of sexual liberation, bizarre fashion, music festivals, student riots and an increase in the availability of illegal substances. According to Conger (1991) no era of history 'contained as many shocks to the sense of cultural order' as did the mid 1960s to the early 1970s.

The previously held views of adolescence only began to be challenged during the 1980s and 1990s when recognition was given to the individual rather than generalizing from the minority. Hauser *et al.* (1991) suggest that, whilst adolescence can be disturbing for both the adolescence and the family, neither respond homogenously to their experiences. The view of storm and stress, turmoil and declining morals has been grossly 'exaggerated' according to Graham and Rutter (1985), and the problems of a few have been applied *en masse* to all who fit the criteria of adolescents. A more accurate assessment might be that a minority of adolescents do engage in behaviour which can be defined as 'rebellious' (Steinberg 1987), and there does appear to be an increase in vandalism and violence, although such activities are by no means solely confined to adolescents. Sexual activity is also clearly likely to increase with age, but again there is little evidence to suggest that all adolescents are promiscuous (see Chapter 8). The greatest problems during adolescence do appear to relate to mood, and Steinberg (1987) suggests that a third to a half of all adolescents experience periods of sadness, anxiety and muddled feelings. Again, such feelings are also experienced by others who would not be classed as adolescents and such statistics ignore the importance of coping mechanisms employed by adolescents which help them deal with such feelings. Whilst we are not denying that adolescents may at times feel sad, for example, we feel it is important to recognize the resilience which the majority of adolescents show in response to negative emotion. Some excellent novels which illustrate this resilience include Françoise Sagan's *Bonjour Tristesse* (1954), Anne Frank's Diary (Frank 1947), Mary Macarthy's *The Group* (1966) and Sue Towsend's *The Secret Diary of Adrian Mole* (1984).

The reasons why adults still, albeit to a lesser extent, carry negative images of adolescence is both puzzling and without doubt can lead to stereotyping and prejudice. Several factors have been identified by Greene and Larson (1991) as exacerbating these negative views of adolescence:

- the over reliance on adult informants and adult-based paradigms;
- the perception of adolescence as an undifferentiated transition to adulthood; and
- insufficient attention to the developmental transitions that both characterize and differentiate adolescence.

Recognizing adolescents as individuals who are undergoing great biological, psychological and social change, who are neither large children, nor small adults, and who require special understanding because of the complex feelings they are experiencing, will hopefully in time remove what has long become a stigma involving a large percentage of the population. Each generation of adults has always found something about adolescence which is perceived to be shocking. In reality, it is probably the difference in behaviour, clothes, language and opportunity which adults find difficult to accept, rather than a lowering of actual moral standards or behaviour. Respecting the right for difference is, we would suggest, a vital prerequisite for nursing these young people.

The implications for nurses

The implications of the previous discussion for nurses are many. Adolescence is difficult to define and, although we would encourage hospitals to develop policies in relation to the care of adolescents, we would suggest that guidance which involves defining adolescence should be fairly fluid to allow for individual differences in development. Nor should policy take only one criterion to define adolescence but should be flexible in approach.

We are clearly left after this discussion with several questions relating to adolescence which we hope the rest of this book will help to clarify. These pertain to the very nature of adolescence and traditional views of the characteristics of this group of individuals. The important thing to remember perhaps is that they are individual and as such are deserving of an individual approach from those who care for them in whatever capacity. The view of adolescence as a time of considerable conflict should not influence our perception or colour our views. Generalizing the problems of a few is, we would suggest, a dangerous practice and opposes the concept of individualized care.

References

Audit Commission (1993) *Children First: A Study of Hospital Services.* HMSO, London.

Blair, G.M., Jones, R.S., and Simpson, R.H. (1962) *Educational Psychology*, 2nd edn. The Macmillan Co., New York.

Booth, B. (1994) A guiding act? *Nursing Times*, 90(8): 30–31.

British Medical Association (1961) *Medical and Social Aspects of Adolescence.* BMA, London.

Burman, D. (1985) The paediatrician and the adolescent. In: NAWCH Report, *Too Old, Too Young.* NAWCH, London.

Buskist, W. and Gerbing, D.W. (1990) *Psychology: Boundaries and Frontiers.* Scott Foresman/Little, Brown, Glenview, Illinois.

Conger, J.J. (1991) *Adolescence and Youth*, 4th edn. Harper Collins, New York.

Court, S.D.M. (1976) *Fit For the Future: Report of the Committee on Child Health Services* Vols I and II. HMSO, London.

Cox, C. (1983) *Sociology: An Introduction for Nurses, Midwives and Health Visitors.* Butterworths, London.

Crehan, K. (1992) Rural households: survival and change. In: *Rural Livelihoods: Crisis and Response.* (Eds H. Bernstein, B. Crow and H. Johnson). Oxford University Press in association with the Open University, Oxford.

Department of Health (1989) *The Children Act.* HMSO, London.

Department of Health (1991) *The Welfare of Children and Young People in Hospital.* HMSO, London.

Dimond, B. (1990) *Legal Aspects of Nursing.* Prentice Hall, New York.

Eppel, E.M. and Eppel, M. (1966) *Adolescents and Morality.* Routledge and Kegan Paul, London.

Erikson, E. (1965) *Childhood and Society.* Penguin, Harmondsworth.

Filpovic, Z. (1994) *Zlata's Diary.* Viking, London.

Frank, A. (1947) *Anne Frank's Diary.* Valentine, Mitchell and Co., London.

Freud, A. (1958) Adolescence. *Psychoanalytic Study of the Child*, 13: 255–278.

Gesell, A., Ilg, F.L., and Bates Ames, L. (1956) *Youth: The Years from Ten to Sixteen.* Hamish Hamilton, London.

Giddens, A. (1989) *Sociology*. Polity Press, Cambridge.

Graham, P. and Rutter, M. (1985) Adolescent disorders. In: *Child and Adolescent Psychiatry: Modern Approaches*, 2nd edn. (Eds M. Rutter and L. Hersov). Blackwell Scientific Publications, Oxford.

Greene, A.L. and Larson, R.W. (1991) Variation in stress reactivity during adolescence. In: *Life-Span Developmental Psychology: Perspectives on Stress and Coping*. (Eds E.M. Cummings, A.L. Greene and K.H. Karraker). Lawrence Erlbaum Associates, Hillsdale, New Jersey.

Gunn, A. (1970) *The Privileged Adolescent*. MTP Press, Lancaster.

Hadfield, J.A. (1962) *Childhood and Adolescence*. Penguin, Harmondsworth.

Hall, G. (1904) *Adolescence: Its Psychology and its Relations to Physiology, Anthropology, Sociology, Sex, Crime, Religion and Education*, Vol I. Prentice-Hall, New Jersey.

Hauser, S., Borman, E., Bowlds, M.K., Powers, S., Jacobson, A., Noam, G. and Knoebber, K. (1991) Understanding coping within adolescence: Ego development and coping strategies. In: *Life-Span Developmental Psychology: Perspectives on Stress and Coping*. (Eds E.M. Cummings, A.L. Greene and K.H. Karraker). Lawrence Erlbaum Associates, Hillsdale, New Jersey.

Hewitt, T. (1992) Children, abandonment and public action. In: *Rural Livelihoods: Crisis and Response*. (Eds H. Bernstein, B. Crow and H. Johnson). Oxford University Press in Association with the Open University, Oxford.

Huchesson, P. (1992) NLJ Law Reports. *New Law Journal*, August 7: 1123–1127.

Jordan, D. and Kelfer, L.S. (1983) Adolescent potential for participation in health care. *Issues in Comprehensive Paediatric Nursing*, 6: 147–156.

Kuykendall, J. (1989) Teenage trauma. *Nursing Times*, 85(27): 26–28.

Macarthy, M. (1966) *The Group*. Penguin, Harmondsworth.

Marcia, J.E. (1982) Identity in adolescence. In: *Handbook of Adolescent Psychology*. (Ed. J. Anderson). John Wiley, Chichester.

Overton, W.F., Ward, S.L., Noveck, I.A., Black, J. and O'Brien, D.P. (1987) Form and content in the development of deductive reasoning. *Developmental Psychology*, 23: 22–30.

Piaget, J. (1954) *The Construction of Reality in the Child*. Basic Books, New York.

Platt, H., Chairman (1959) *The Welfare of Children in Hospital: Report of the Committee on Child Health Services*. (*The Platt Report*). HMSO, London.

Rutter, M. (1979) *Changing Youth in a Changing Society: Patterns of Adolescent Development and Disorder*. The Nuffield Provincial Hospitals Trust, London.

Sagan, F. (1954) *Bonjour Tristesse*. Julliard, Paris.

Shield, J.P.H. and Baum, J.D. (1994) Children's consent to treatment. *British Medical Journal*, 308: 1182–1183.

Steinberg, D. (1987) *Basic Adolescent Psychiatry*. Blackwell Scientific Publications, Oxford.

Swanwick, M. (1990) Knowledge and control. *Paediatric Nursing*, 2(5): 18–20.

Townsend, S. (1984) *The Secret Diary of Adrian Mole Aged 13¾*. Methuen, London.

United States Department of Health, Welfare and Education (1979) *Adolescent Health Care: A Guide for BCHS-Supported Programs and Projects.* DHEW, Washington.

Windmill, V. (1987) *Human Growth and Development.* Edward Arnold, London.

World Health Organization (1977) *Health Needs of Adolescents* (WHO Expert Committee Technical Report Series 609). WHO, Geneva.

Further reading

Brazier, M (1992) *Medicine, Patients and the Law,* new edn. Penguin Harmondsworth.

Chapter 15 of this book relates to doctors and child patients, giving an account of relevant law in the area of consent.

Dimond, B. (1990) *Legal Aspects of Nursing.* Prentice Hall, New York.

This text also explores legal aspects of nursing minors.

Chapter 2
Family Relationships

Adolescence is a period during which young people strive to become relatively independent from their parents. The family are usually extremely influential in this process. The degree of problem solving experience afforded to the adolescent, the level of authority within the family context and a number of other variables, will in many ways shape the process and outcome of gaining independence.

Parent–child relationships prior to adolescence will also affect how parents and adolescents interact and communicate. For example, children who have been over protected, possibly due to chronic ill health, may find it difficult as adolescents to cope with the demands of being independent. Essential adult skills of problem solving and decision making are clearly not ours by right. These skills develop throughout childhood and adolescence, and require both experience and practice. Over-protected children may be denied the opportunity of practising such skills, of making mistakes and of learning through those mistakes, and may find independence and the demands that it brings, a traumatic experience.

For nurses involves in the care of adolescents who are well or sick a knowledge of family dynamics is extremely important in understanding adolescent behaviour. Prior and current parent–adolescent interaction will influence health and illness behaviour, health beliefs and health knowledge. This chapter will therefore explore the influence of the family on the process of gaining independence and health behaviour.

The changing structure and status of the family

It is not the intention here to give a detailed sociological account of the changing nature of the family. There are many good sociology texts for nurses which can give such detail (see Further reading). What we do wish to do is to explore how changes in the status and structure of the family across time have impacted upon adolescent development, and to discuss how different family structures which exist within any given society may influence adolescent autonomy and independence.

Extended families

In pre-industrial Britain the typical family structure was the 'extended family', with large family groups, consisting of parents, grandparents, children, aunts, uncles, cousins and other related kin living in close proximity to each other. This type of family structure is not by any means extinct and such family groups can be seen today in both developed and developing countries.

The importance of the extended family upon adolescent development is a largely unexplored area. However, certain influences of growing up in close proximity to a large family network are evident. First of all, families will function according to a family code (Sameroff 1989) which regulates development to produce family members who fulfil a role within the family and who can participate in shared activity. Parents also have a parenting code which has a similar influence within small nuclear families. Adolescents growing up as part of an extended family network will be influenced by parenting codes, and by family codes. They are able to observe vicariously the effects of conforming to codes, and breaking codes. To a large extent parenting codes will be influenced by family codes. However, when adolescents may feel confused about parenting codes, the family code provides a stable and readily available guide.

Secondly, the extended family provides a group of close adult role models, apart from parents, who the adolescent can observe. (Of course, this may not always be a positive feature.) Adult and close-age members of the extended family can not only provide a guide for behaviour, but also can assist in the learning of coping behaviours and problem solving strategies.

Thirdly, extended families can provide an informal social support network which can help the nuclear family function both under normal situations and under stress. Adolescents, in particular female adolescents, in isolated distressed nuclear families may have to assume a 'pseudoparenting' role (Greene and Larson 1991), whereas families living in close proximity to extended families usually have other adult members who can provide necessary support which can minimize adolescent stress and overall family distress.

The nuclear family

Although extended family networks do exist in Britain, particularly in rural locations and among certain cultural groups, there has been a distinct trend since the industrial revolution towards nuclear family structures. These family structures consist of parents and children, living in geographic isolation from the extended family. They tend to be relatively mobile structures, and adult females are more likely to be in paid employment outside the home.

The influence of the isolated nuclear family upon the developing adolescent might initially appear to be negative in comparison to the extended family network, and clearly there are certain disadvantages. The overall influence cannot however be all negative, since most of us now grow up within such structures and survive. In terms of adolescent autonomy and independence, growing up within a nuclear family which in itself is independent from wider family structures can be positive and advantageous. Families have to develop ways of problem solving and coping which do not rely on close family social support. Where parents cope successfully in isolation, clearly they provide positive role models for adolescents who are learning to develop their own coping strategies. Hauser *et al.* (1991) suggest that the diverse ways in which adolescents learn to cope are influenced by individual and contextual factors, such as:

'the family setting, including continuing relationships with parents, availability of parents, past identification with parents, and the presence of parents as role models, in dyadic and familial interactions' (p178).

A further advantage of growing up in an isolated nuclear family relates to adolescent choice, particularly in relation to vocation. Extended families living in close proximity tended to remain close because of shared male employment and patrilineal inheritance. Children, particularly male children would have little choice about vocation. This type of restricted choice can be seen today in developing countries (Crehan 1992), and among certain occupational groups in developed countries. For example, in farming communities in rural Britain large extended families still exist, with male (and female) adolescents following their parents' vocation. Adolescents in isolated nuclear families arguably have greater choice about how their adult lives will be structured although, realistically, high unemployment is limiting choice to some extent. Greater educational opportunity and a lack of geographic restriction however do potentially allow adolescents from isolated nuclear families greater flexibility.

Divorce, one-parent families and re-structured families

In this chapter so far we have focused on parents and adolescents living either near or apart from their extended family. Clearly, the view that adolescents will grow up with *two* parents, or if they do that they will be *biological* parents is outmoded and unrealistic. The increase in the number of divorces, more frequent remarriage and greater social acceptability towards having children outside marriage has had a major influence on family structures. Just as adolescents in isolated nuclear families are less likely to have contact with extended kin, so many adolescents grow up having very limited or no contact with one biological parent.

The effects of divorce and of growing up in a single parent or reconstituted family are varied. Studies suggest that boys are more adversely affected than girls by divorce particularly in relation to academic measures (Hetherington 1989), and Wolkind and Rutter (1985) suggest that teachers respond less positively to male children from divorced families. Wolkind and Rutter also suggest that boys show less social affiliation and greater social isolation. That is not to say that girls are not affected by divorce. Indeed both boys and girls do suffer profound effects (Guidubaldi *et al.* 1986), although Forchand *et al.* (1991) suggest that effects are more pronounced during pre-adolescence than during the adolescent years.

The reasons for age differences in the impact of divorce upon children is unclear but probably reflect wider life experience and problem solving skill. Wolkind and Rutter (1985) suggest that adolescents whose parents have divorced show a wide range of coping abilities and strategies. A not infrequent strategy involves detachment from parental problems with increased interaction outside the home. Conger (1991) suggests however that divorce can impact upon adolescents' abilities to form relationships of their own, implying that adolescents are wary of intimate relationships *per se*, and cope with their wariness by not putting themselves in a position which could cause them stress. It is difficult though to measure whether this is a reaction to the divorce itself or whether, for example, marital disharmony prior to divorce is significant. Marital disharmony usually precedes divorce making it difficult to differentiate between these two variables. Studies of children and adolescents who witness marital disharmony outside divorce suggest that it does, on its own have adverse psychological effects particularly when disharmony includes violence (Bennett 1991; Rossman and Rosenberg 1992).

Clearly, marital disharmony is only one of a number of variables which affect how children and adolescents are influenced by divorce. These include the degree of emotional distress, changes in lifestyle after the divorce and the involvement of parents in intimate relationships with other adults (see Wolkind and Rutter 1985 for a review). Growing up in a one-parent family is also an increasing phenomenon, partially due to the increase in divorce but also attributable to an increase in the numbers of women who have children outside marriage. Conger (1991) suggests that 90% of one-parent families in the USA comprise of a mother and one or more children. Similar trends are evident in Britain. Paternal absence is then something which many young people will experience. The effect of growing up without a father has been the subject of some investigation which indicates that there are differences between boys and girls in terms of psychological impact. Fry and Scher's (1984) longitudinal study is of particular interest in that it identified a growing trend towards decline in achievement motivation in boys during early and middle adolescence. However, as with the effects of divorce, the younger the age at which boys lose their fathers the more likely they are to experience adverse psychological effects. Clearly, also, the personality of the mother and the presence of other adult males are variables which may limit negative outcome at any age. Further work has concentrated on the influence of father absence on psychosexual development in boys. Wolkind and Rutter (1985) suggest that links between father absence and homosexuality, however, should be treated with caution.

'Clearly the crude stereotype that the lack of a father leads to homosexuality or femininity in boys can be rejected' (p48).

The influence of father absence on girls is vastly under researched and recent empirical work is sadly lacking. The paucity of research is disappointing particularly in view of the numbers of female children and adolescents who live in mother-only environments. Data relating to maternal absence are also limited although, as with children growing up in mother-only families, the personality of the present father and the degree of social support are limiting factors. One interesting study however does highlight the potential problems which fathers may face in terms of interaction with professionals, and clearly this study has relevance to health care professionals. Fry and Addington (1984) asked a sample of social workers, teachers and lay people to make judgements on the basis of watching a videotape of four 10-year-old boys. A third of the sample were told that the boys lived in father-absent homes, a third were told that the boys lived in mother-absence homes and the remaining third were told the boys came from intact homes. The results showed that the subjects who were told that the boys were from mother-absence homes judged the boys to be less happy, less emotionally adjusted and more delinquent than did the other two groups of subjects. It is interesting to note that these judgement were as evident among the teachers and social workers in the sample as among lay subjects. It would be particularly interesting to replicate this study some ten years on and to include nurses and other clinical health professionals in the sample.

For many children and adolescents living in one-parent households is a temporary state. Re-structured families, which include the presence of an adult who is not biologically related, are increasingly common. Such re-structured families may or may not include other children who are not biologically related, or who are half-siblings. The effects of living in a re-structured family depend largely upon communication and interaction within the new family and the child's relationship with the absent parent (Conger 1991). Previous experiences prior to the constitution of the new family are obviously pivotal to the success or otherwise of adaptation to a re-structured family. It is interesting to note, however, that boys appear to adapt less well than girls – particularly if they were nine years or older when their mothers remarried (see Wolkind and Rutter 1985). Younger boys were able to develop good relationships with their stepfathers.

We suggested at the beginning of this section that the concept of children growing up with two biological parents was unrealistic but perhaps society's continued focus on this 'ideal family' could in part be detrimental to children and adolescents who grow up in one-parent or re-structured families. Children do not like to appear different and some of the psychopathology observed in such children could be attributable to their own perceptions of what is normal and what is not. Wise (1994) in her work on the changing face of the family writes:

'The concept of the two-parent, two-child family as the norm is a myth, and probably always has been a myth; nevertheless, it is this mythical family that is used as the basis for policy making, and that tends to be the family structure of expectation. Families come in all shapes and sizes, and it is the 'whole' that is important, rather than the sum of the parts' (p39).

Perhaps if less emphasis was placed on the norm and a more realistic view of the contemporary family was adopted by policy makers, the media, schools, health services etc. then children and adolescents who are not from 'ideal' families may feel better about themselves. There is clearly scope for further research into these issues, particularly in relation to *why* children and adolescents experience difficulties and *what* society can do to help them.

Models of parenting

So far we have discussed the types of family structure which commonly exist in Britain, and how these structures may influence the lives of adolescents. We now move on to look at variations in family relationships which have relevance regardless of family structure. There are a number of ways of classifying different types of family relationships. Powers *et al.* (1983) proposed what is probably the simplest classification, describing family relationships as being 'enabling' or not, in terms of the way that the family system promotes adolescent autonomy and independence. The reasons why families are, or are not enabling are eloquently reviewed by Sameroff (1989), who discusses the importance of not only recognizing that parents are the 'major regulatory agency' in terms of child development, but also that parental behaviour is 'embedded in regulatory contexts'.

These regulatory contexts occur at three levels. The first level is referred to as 'macroregulation'. Macroregulations are culturally derived regulations which dictate the basis of socialization within each culture. For example, adolescents must attend school until they reach the age of 16 in Britain, and fasting during the month of Ramadan is compulsory for all Muslims who have reached puberty. Clearly these macroregulations influence parental behaviour, and ultimately adolescent experiences.

The second regulatory level is referred to as 'miniregulation' which whilst still conforming to cultural codes, reflects more the day-to-day interaction which occurs between parents and their children. For example, families develop their own individual ways of disciplining children but normally do so within culturally defined boundaries. Miniregulations observed in parents often reflect the family codes by which they themselves have been reared, particularly in extended family systems. Children and adolescents learn to interact according to the family's own miniregulations, and also recognize the consequences of not doing so. They can also be instrumental, particularly as they grow older, in shaping family miniregulations.

The third level of regulation is referred to as 'microregulation'. This occurs at an individual level between members of the family and is influenced by individual characteristics such as personality and temperament. Microregulations tend to be brief interactions which appear to occur spontaneously but which, when the two interacting family members are attuned to each other, can regulate behaviour. For example, an adolescent may stop behaving in a certain way in response to a slight change in a parent's facial expression or body posture.

The three regulatory levels are important in determining patterns of parenting, and in understanding variations in adolescent–parent interaction which will be discussed in the next section. It is also important for nurses to recognize that adolescent and parental behaviour are both intertwined and regulated by cultural and family contexts as well as individual predispositions.

The processes by which regulation takes place involve the way that parents communicate, provide emotional support and exert control upon children and adolescents. Baumrind (1967) provided a basis for classifying parenting patterns in relation to regulatory roles, by studying small groups of nursery school children. She concluded that parenting patterns could influence child behaviour and identified three types of children. The first group of children were described by Baumrind as being well adjusted, and their parents were typically warm, nurturing, supportive and controlling. The second group of children were defined as being insecure and apprehensive. Baumrind identified that their parents were also controlling, but were less nurturing and had a tendency to frighten children. Her findings suggest that parents of insecure children are not more controlling, but that they exert control without emotional support. The third group of children were described as aggressive and impulsive. Their parents were more likely to be less controlling, less demanding and less well organized than parents of children in the other two groups.

Based on Baumrind's findings, parenting patterns have been commonly categorized as being 'authoritative', 'authoritarian' or 'permissive'. Clearly not all parenting patterns will fit exclusively into one of these categories just as not all children and adolescents will fit into one or other of Baumrind's child classifications. However, the parenting patterns do provide a useful model for considering family dynamics.

Authoritative parenting

Authoritative parents also demand high levels of control, but combine that control with warmth, emotional support and rationale for setting limits to behave. Communication and interaction levels are high. This type of parenting style elicits the most positive outcomes in terms of child and adolescent behaviour (Bee 1992). Adolescents from authoritative families are likely to exhibit higher self-esteem and will generally accept, rather than reject, parental control because parents make it clear that control is based on a rational concern for the young person's welfare (Conger 1991). In Burbach's study (1989) adolescents from authoritative families were less likely to demonstrate psychopathology.

Authoritarian parenting

Typically authoritarian parents demand high levels of control with low levels of warmth or emotional support. Authoritarian parents expect obedience without giving explanation as to why obedience is desirable. Adolescents are expected to comply without question, because of parental conviction that they are right. Negotiation is not part of the agenda. Adolescents from authoritarian families typically have lowered self-esteem, and a study by Burbach *et al..* (1989) which compared parenting patterns among a group of adolescents identified that depressed adolescents were more likely than non-depressed adolescents to have authoritarian parents.

Permissive parenting

The third type of parenting patterns concerns permissive or *laissez-faire* parents. These parents attempt to exert little control over adolescents and may wish to adopt the role of peer rather than parent. They find it difficult to act as a figure of authority. Adolescents from permissive families tend to be more aggressive than their peers, and less willing to take responsibility (Conger 1991), possibly because parental role models shun responsibility themselves. They are also less likely to be independent than their peers. It appears that several factors may be involved in the poor outcome relating to this type of parenting. First of all adolescents want their parents to be parents and not their equals. Secondly that concern for welfare and emotional support appears to enable the adolescent to easily identify boundaries for behaviour. Without such support behaviour appears to be more erratic and controlled. Finally, adolescents appear to need a role model in their parent who is both responsible and independent.

Independence from parents

The increased independence which is a major task of adolescence has been the focus of a great deal of speculation. Freud, for example, saw adolescence as a period during which the previously held identification with the same sex parent is weakened and renewed identification with the opposite sex parent occurs. Later work by psychologists from the psychoanalytical school expanded on this work and sought to explain the process by which adolescents became independent from both parents, and replaced family ties by engaging in group activities, by getting involved in exciting experiences, and by becoming involved in frequent and abrupt relationships (see Gross 1992). Gaining independence must however be viewed within both cultural and familial contexts, which evidently influence this process.

This chapter has taken as its main focus family interaction and how adolescents seek to gain independence from the family. Clearly there are many factors which will influence the extent to which independence is achieved and the ease with which independence occurs. Family structure, regulation within the family, parenting patterns and other factors such as cultural and socioeconomic status are all variables which will influence the process of gaining independence during adolescence. This process must be viewed as a two-way interaction. First of all it involves the extent to which adolescents are prepared for, and motivated towards, independence, and secondly, it involves parental willingness to allow and facilitate adolescent independence. This willingness is influenced by many factors which have been discussed throughout this chapter. However, when adolescents are ill, particularly if they have a chronic and persisting health problem, the process of gaining independence is subject to further complex variables.

Adolescents with health problems – gaining independence

The extent to which adolescents who have health problems are able to gain independence from the family is to some extent dependent on two inter-related factors. The first of these relates to the previous experiences of the adolescent and family during sickness. Most children experience minor illnesses during their early years, and Parmalee (1986) suggests that the way early, minor illness is handled within the family is important in terms of dealing with more severe illness later on. Parental confidence, for example, can be severely affected by early adverse experiences. Parmalee (1989) further highlights this point:

> 'how parents and children cope emotionally and cognitively with major acute illnesses is, in part, a function of how successful they have been in dealing with minor physical disturbances that have previously occurred' (p149).

Early experiences can then determine a family's style in dealing with major illness during adolescence and the degree of independence awarded to adolescents who are ill. Young people who have health problems may have their activity limited or facilitated by parents and other family members. Talcott Parsons (1951) described the concept of the 'sick role' which is accorded to sick individuals and excludes them from carrying out their usual daily activities. Each family will have its own version of the sick role and adolescents learn early on their own family's version, which can influence their own understanding of illness and its consequences. The family can be highly influential, for example, in persuading an adolescent who is feeling moderately unwell that a day off school is a sensible option – the doctor is called and the young person is put to bed.

The second factor which can influence the degree of independence afforded or gained by adolescents relates to the nature of illness. Some adolescents may be dependent upon parents for physiotherapy or medication, for example, which may limit activity. There may, however, be marked differences in the perceptions of parents and adolescents about the degree of dependence required (Dragone 1990), and sensitive intervention by health care professionals may alleviated conflict. Adolescents can successfully be taught self-care which will enable greater independence (Dryden 1989). In the United States, summer camps organized for children and adolescents with specific health problems, and staffed by medically trained workers can introduce adolescents to safe independence, and allow parents to 'let go' whilst knowing that if problems occur there are people on hand who will cope. Such camps are becoming more popular in Britain and offer many advantages to young people with chronic health problems. Not only do they allow peer interaction with people who have similar experiences, they also allow the adolescent to gain confidence in coping ability and promote independence.

The implications for nurses

The importance of nurses understanding family dynamics cannot be underestimated. Adolescents, whether well or sick, are still heavily influenced by parents and family. Parents and families are in turn heavily influenced by adolescent behaviour.

It is perhaps somewhat obvious to emphasize that health care professionals need to be aware that adolescents may come from families which do not include two biological parents. It is however all too easy to make inaccurate assumptions, particularly in the absence of detailed information. Many nurses have recounted experiences of absent biological parents not being informed that a child is ill or has had an accident, and of the intense guilt and blame which absent and present parents can experience. The importance of enquiring sensitively about the family structure cannot be over estimated. One-parent families with younger children may, for example, need tangible support in order to spend time with an adolescent in hospital.

It is also important that nurses are aware of their own potential prejudices and how these may affect their perception of adolescents. We have mentioned the study by Fry and Addington (1984) and recommend that nurses should explore not only their attitudes towards mother-absent families, but also towards other alternative family structures. Exploring and understanding cultural and family codes, and family regulatory systems should also form part of the nursing assessment. There are cultural differences both within and across countries and such exploration will facilitate the development of a therapeutic relationship, and may enable the nurse to gain insight into adolescent–parental interaction. So too is it important to recognize parenting patterns which may influence adolescent behaviour. Clearly when adolescents are required to make decisions, possibly regarding health care, parenting patterns may effect both adolescents' willingness to take responsibility for their own health, and parent's willingness to allow the adolescent choice.

We have also discussed parenting patterns which may affect how adolescents and parents interact during periods of ill health and in relation to how the adolescent makes health choices. The authoritarian parents who dictate that an adolescent should 'do as he is told' pose several problems for health care professionals and possibly for the adolescent. So too can the permissive parent who seems to care little for what the adolescent does or says. The effect of parenting patterns on adolescent behaviour can be marked and nurses should be aware of the potential influence upon adolescent behaviour. The overt attitude observed in an adolescent may well be more attributable to parenting patterns than to personality or temperament.

Finally, we have discussed how illness may affect the adolescent's degree of independence and clearly it is important that nurses should explore with adolescents and their families their perceptions of illness and dependence. Careful intervention can assist the adolescent in becoming more independent, by for example teaching adolescents how to perform medical procedures such as passing nasogastric tubes on themselves. Finding out about opportunities offered by various organizations for holidays may also enable adolescents and their parents to consider alternatives to restrictive dependence.

References

Baumrind, D. (1967) Childcare practices anteceding three patterns of pre-school behaviour. *Genetic Psychology Monographs*, 735: 43–88.

Bee, H. (1992) *The Developing Child*, 6th edn. Harper Collins, New York.

Bennett, L. (1991) Adolescent girls' experience of witnessing marital violence: a phenomenological study. *Journal of Advanced Nursing*, 16: 431–438.

Burbach, D.J., Kashani, J.H. and Rosenberg, T.K. (1989) Parental bonding and depressive disorders in adolescents. *Journal of Child Psychology and Psychiatry*, 30(3): 417–429.

Conger, J.J. (1991) *Adolescence and Youth: Psychological Development in a Changing World*. Harper Collins, New York.

Crehan, K. (1992) Rural households: survival and change. In: *Rural Livelihoods: Crisis and Response.* (Eds H. Bernstein, B. Crow and H. Johnson). Oxford University Press in association with the Open University, Oxford.

Dragone, M.A. (1990) Perspectives of chronically ill adolescents and parents on health care needs. *Paediatric Nursing,* 16(1), 45–50.

Dryden, S. (1989) Paediatric medicine in the community. *Paediatric Nursing,* 1(8): 17–18.

Forchand, R., Neighbors, B. and Wierson, M. (1991) The transition to adolescence: the role of gender and stress in problem behavior and competence. *Journal of Child Psychology and Psychiatry,* 32(6): 929–937.

Fry, P.S. and Addington, J. (1984) Professionals' negative expectations of boys from father headed single-parent families: implications for the training of child-care professionals. *British Journal of Developmental Psychology,* 2: 337–346.

Fry, P.S. and Scher, A. (1984) The effect of father absence on children's motivation, ego-strength, and locus of control orientation: a five year longitudinal assessment. *British Journal of Developmental Psychology,* 2: 167–168.

Greene, A.L. and Larson, R.N. (1991) Variations in stress reactivity during adolescence. In: *Life Span Developmental Psychology: Perspectives on Stress and Coping.* (Eds. E.M. Cummings, A.L. Greene and K.H. Karraker). Lawrence Erlbaum Associates, New Jersey.

Gross, R.D. (1992) *Psychology: The Science of Mind and Behaviour,* 2nd edn. Hodder and Stoughton, London.

Guidubaldi, J., Cleminshaw, H.K., Perry, J.D., Natasi, B.K. and Lichtel, J. (1986) The role of selected environment factors in children's post-divorce adjustment. *Family Relationships,* 35: 141–151.

Hauser, S., Borman, E., Bowlds, M.K., Powers, S., Jacobson, A., Noam, G. and Knoebber, K. (1991) Understanding coping within adolescence: ego development and coping strategies. In: *Life Span Developmental Psychology: Perspectives on Stress and Coping.* (Eds E.M. Cummings, A.L. Greene and K.H. Karraker). Lawrence Erlbaum Associates, New Jersey.

Hetherington, E.M. (1989) Coping with family transitions: winners, losers and survivors. *Child Development,* 60, 1–14.

Parmalee, A.H. (1986) Children's illnesses: their beneficial effects on their behavioural development. *Child Development,* 57: 1–10.

Parmalee, A.H. (1989) The child's physical health and the development of relationships. In: *Relationship Disturbances in Early Childhood: A Developmental Approach.* Basic Books, New York.

Parsons, T. (1951) *The Social System.* Free Press, Illinois.

Powers, S., Hauser, S., Schwartz, J., Noam, G. and Jacobson, A. (1983) Adolescent ego development and family interaction. In: *Adolescent Development in the Family.* (Eds H. Grotevant and C. Cooper). Jossey Bass, San Francisco.

Rossman, B.B.R. and Rosenberg, M.S. (1992) Family stress and functioning in children: the moderating effects of children's beliefs about their control over parental conflict. *Journal of Child Psychology and Psychiatry,* 33(4): 699–716.

Sameroff, A.J. (1989) Principles of development and psychopathology. In: *Relationship Disturbances in Early Childhood: A Developmental Approach.* (Eds A.J. Sameroff and R.N. Emde). Basic Books, New York.

Wise, G. (1994) The changing family. In: *The Child and Family: Contemporary Nursing Issues in Child Health and Care.* (Ed. B. Lindsay). Baillière Tindall, London.

Wolkind, S. and Rutter, M. (1985) Separation, loss and family relationships. In: *Child and Adolescent Psychiatry: Modern Approaches*, 2nd edn. (Eds M. Rutter and L. Hersov). Blackwell Scientific Publications, Oxford.

Further reading

Haralambos, M. and Holborn, M. (1991) *Sociology: Themes and Perspectives*, 3rd edn. Collins Educational, London.

Chapter 8, which explores families and households, makes interesting reading. In this chapter changes to the family are discussed as well as alternatives to the family.

Sameroff, A.J. and Emde, R.N. (eds) (1989) *Relationship Disturbance in Early Childhood: A Developmental Approach.* Basic Books, New York.

This well written and intriguing text explores the many factors which contribute to the psychological development of the child.

Chapter 3
Individual Differences in Development

One of the most fascinating aspects of adolescence is the variation which occurs between individuals in terms of both physiological growth and psychological development. Variations can also be observed between male and female adolescents and between individuals from different cultural groups. These differences are important for both the adolescents themselves and also for nurses who are involved with their care. Nurses cannot make assumptions about the relationship between chronological age and psychosocial functioning at this, more than at any other stage during the human lifespan. Physical appearance and age, as we will see in this chapter, are poor determinants of understanding and ability. This chapter will therefore focus on the individual differences between adolescents and those factors which influence the rate and outcome of development. It will include exploration of physical development, the changing nature of peer relationships, and discussion regarding psychosocial development. An understanding of these concepts is an important part of being able to engage in appropriate levels of interaction with individual adolescents, particularly in relation to the assessment of individual need.

Physiological development

Adolescence is a period which is marked by rapid physiological growth and development. An increase in gonadotrophin from the pituitary gland results in the stimulation of the testes to produce testosterone in boys, and the stimulation of the ovaries to produce oestrogen in girls. Testicular growth is usually complete between the ages of 13 and 17 years in boys, whereas oestrogen production in girls starts to undergo cyclical changes at around the time of menarche, which usually occurs between 10 and 16 years (Graham and Rutter 1985).

These primary characteristics are clearly important in the lives of adolescents, but it is the development of the secondary sexual characteristics which are most significant in terms of their effect upon appearance. The development of breasts in girls is one of the early characteristics of puberty, both sexes grow pubic and axillary hair, and an increase in the size and secretions of the sebaceous follicles, can lead to the development of skin blemishes in both sexes (Vaughan and Litt 1990).

Further physical changes also occur. The adolescent 'growth spurt' is an early sign of puberty in girls, who also show an increase in hip width. In boys the increase in height is a later manifestation of puberty. They also tend to lose body fat and develop shoulder width. As height velocity slows down, a rapid rise in body fat occurs. These changes can be extremely distressing to adolescents and can lead to feelings of being out of control, although Graham and Rutter (1985) suggest that boys tend to welcome the physical changes whereas girls do not. It is therefore not surprising, for example, that adolescence is the most likely time for eating disorders to develop (Agras and Kirkley 1986), particularly among girls (see Chapter 7). Boys commonly report feeling 'gangly', with limbs appearing too long in relation to the rest of their bodies.

Early and late development

The variations between individuals in terms of the development of primary and secondary characteristics are immense. Very early or late

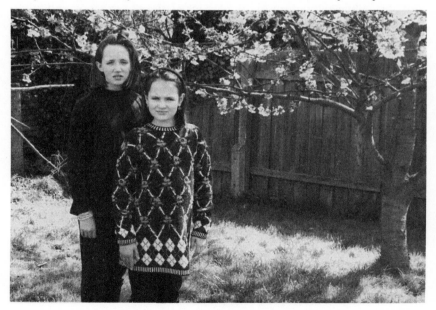

Fig. 3.1 Individual differences can be marked, as these 13-year-old first cousins show: the smaller girl is three months older than her cousin.

development can be distressing to some adolescents as they compare themselves with their more average-looking peers (Adams 1983), and with the stereotypical ideals as portrayed by the media. The individual's perception of what constitutes earliness or lateness, however, is probably more crucial than the actual timing of development. Mussen *et al.* (1990) suggest that early or late physical maturation will have greater psychological effects upon boys than girls. They suggest that early maturing boys may feel different from their peers, but will not tend to feel insecure because they can observe their own development towards the socially acceptable norm. They are more likely to be athletic achievers, are more reserved, self-assured and are more likely to engage in socially appropriate behaviour. Late maturing boys, on the other hand, may experience anxiety as to whether they will ever develop physically, or achieve full maturity. As a result they tend to be less poised, more tense and self-conscious, less popular with peers and are less likely to be leaders.

The picture in early and late maturing girls is quite different. Mussen *et al.* (1990), for example, suggest that early maturing girls in the USA tend to be less satisfied with their body image, are moody, less popular with same-sex peers (although more popular with opposite-sex peers), and do less well academically than late maturing girls.

The extent to which psychological differences associated with late and early physical maturation persist into later adolescence and adulthood is interesting, and again gender differences can be observed. The psychological differences between late and early maturing boys are thought to persist into adulthood (Livson and Peskin 1982), whereas in girls the adverse effects of early development tend to disappear, and early maturers emerge as popular with peers of both sexes, and tend to be more self-directed than their later maturing peers.

One explanation for the initial problems experienced by early maturing girls could relate to the cultural stereotypes referred to above. Society views thin as beautiful, and the changes in fat distribution that occur in early maturing girls can appear to take the adolescent girl away from what she considers to be a socially acceptable body shape. Tobin-Richards *et al.* (1984) suggest that early maturing girls *do* tend to be bigger, heavier and fatter than their peers, and Peterson (1987) found that early maturing girls have a tendency to view themselves as fat, even if they are not. Given that adolescent girls who perceive themselves as being fat tend to set themselves apart from their peers because they fear rejection (Tobias and Gordon 1980), it is possible that initial difficulties with their less mature peers may arise from the early maturing girls themselves rather than from their peers. As peers 'catch up', and body shape stabilizes, the early effects are minimized.

The reasons why psychological problems in late maturing boys persist into adulthood are unknown, and clearly warrant further study. A possible reason could again relate to cultural 'norms', which would also account for the gender differences observed. There are various culturally acceptable stereotypes for girls, which range from small, thin and petite through to tall, thin and elegant, whereas for boys there tends only to be the stereotypical tall, athletic ideal. Thus, whereas small girls have an ideal with which they can identify, small boys do not. Further discussion relating to cultural stereotypes and body image can be found in Chapter 7.

Psychological development

The essential psychosocial tasks of adolescence are discussed fully in Chapter 4. It is important however to consider how physical development interacts with psychosocial development, and how these two interrelated facets of development influence important aspects of adolescence such as the formation of peer relationships. Erikson (1965) has made a major impact in this field in suggesting that the psychosocial tasks of adolescence are inherently different from those tasks encountered at any other stage of the lifespan. Childhood identifications need to be replaced by new and more independent identifications as the adolescent develops a sense of identity as a unique person. Erikson thought that a clear sense of identity is a prerequisite of being able to form intimate relationships, although it must be emphasized that Erikson did not see the development of a sense of identity as only occurring during adolescence. The foundations for developing a sense of identity are laid down in childhood, and normally continue into adulthood. Marcia (1982), who has researched extensively into Erikson's work and extended Erikson's theory, suggests that during the search for a sense of identity, most adolescents experience crisis, whereby the adolescent seeks to resolve various issues relating to personal goals and values. The resolution of crisis does not, however, occur within a vacuum, but within the context of relationships, both with the family and with peers.

The need to 'find oneself' is then one of the main psychosocial driving forces of adolescence, and is an important element in directing, and enabling, the adolescent to identify with reference groups. Such reference groups may be overtly identifiable because of their physical appearance (clothes, hairstyle, make-up etc.), whilst others are identifiable because of the activities they engage in (attending church, going to specific musical events etc.). Physical appearance may well be a limiting factor in being able to engage in certain chosen activities, and may

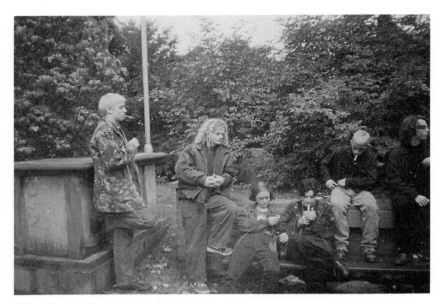

Fig. 3.2   Adolescents need to identify with reference groups.

influence the search for identity, and adolescent feelings of 'belonging'.

Whilst there is little empirical evidence to support the postulate that the rates of physical and psychological development are positively correlated, variations in physical maturation, as discussed in the previous section, certainly appear to influence psychosocial development. Early studies in the United States (see Rutter 1979) suggested, for example, that early maturers, particularly boys, had slight advantages in terms of personality. Although differences found were small, early maturing boys were more popular, more relaxed, more good natured and more poised. Rutter suggested, however, that advantages of early maturation tend to vary according to culture and socioeconomic status, implying that physical development must be viewed within the social context of the individual adolescent.

Cognitive development

The search for a sense of identity as discussed by Erikson (1965) cannot be seen as the whole psychological theory which seeks to explain how adolescents 'find themselves'. The development of identity depends largely upon cognitive abilities, with the adolescent needing to be able to conceptualize, and engage in systematic and rational abstract thinking.

Piaget (1952) (see Chapter 5) has done much to clarify the way cognitive skills develop, and by the identification of discrete cognitive stages enables correlations to be made between cognitive abilities and identity formation. Whilst some of Piaget's work has been criticized, often because his original experiments were complex and his stages over-mechanized, the shift in thinking which occurs sometime after the age of 12 does, to a certain extent, help to explain why adolescents start to question their previous goals and reach out for new and broader horizons. This 'reaching out' process invariably involves a degree of psychological withdrawal from the family, and the seeking of closer reciprocal relationships with peers.

Moral development

Any discussion relating to adolescents 'finding themselves' would be incomplete without reference to moral development, which refers to the development of a person's thoughts and actions about what is right and wrong. Every adolescent will at some time be faced with changing, and sometimes conflicting, values and standards of behaviour, and will inevitably have to make choices about his or her own actions and behaviour (Conger 1991). During adolescence, as at other times during the lifespan, individuals will look towards their reference groups, in order to gain some insight into how they should behave. This process, however, is not as simple as it sounds, and is complicated by the adolescent's lack of experience in making moral decisions, and by the sometimes conflicting views of the individual's reference groups. Conflicting views of parents and peers are, for example, not uncommon as many adolescents and parents will testify!

How adolescents cope with conflict and arrive at their own personal set of guiding norms and beliefs is complex and subject to the influence of several variables including learning within the family group, morals, religious teaching and previous experience. Previous experience at dealing with conflict, decision-making and problem solving skills are also thought to be extremely important. Rest (1986) suggests that the degree of social experience, experience of making decisions, and meeting different types of people will all influence later moral development. Educational experience is also significant, because they enable children to practice problem-solving skills. Just as the search for identity cannot be separated from cognitive development, moral development is thought to be positively correlated with cognitive development. Kohlberg's theory of moral development (see Baskist and Gerring 1990) was partially based on the premise that as children develop cognitively, so they develop morally.

[Handwritten note overlaid on lower right portion of page:]

※ Examples of Panchard.

Adolescent Health Care —

P.51 Ch 4 — Nursing adol.

— Gaining independence from parents — self worth — self esteem

(1)

six stages of moral development and, though his theory has been the subject of some criticism (mainly because much of his experimentation was carried out on male subjects), it is useful in terms of gaining some understanding into adolescent behaviour.

At Level one, which Kohlberg referred to as the 'preconventional level', individuals (usually children, but some adolescents and adults never progress beyond this level) tend to behave in ways which will gain reward and avoid punishment. Their actions are almost wholly determined by the consequences of those actions and they are extremely obedient to authority particularly physically superior authority (e.g. parents, teachers). The individual's standards are almost entirely externally imposed, rather than being internal. Stage 1 and Stage 2 are the stages of the preconventional level, and individuals will move from being selfish, egocentric and obedience oriented, towards taking the views of others into account, if they think they will gain by doing so. For example, a child may give another child one of his sweets if he thinks he'll be given one back.

At Level two, which Kohlberg referred to as 'conventional morality', moral reasoning is again determined partially upon whether others will approve of actions and behaviours, and includes cognisance of rules and laws (Buskist and Gerbing 1990). During Stage 3, the first stage of conventional morality, the individual's behaviour will conform according to the wishes of others, in order to gain approval and feel good about oneself. The individual will also value mutual relationships, and will attempt to look at things from the point of view of others. By Stage 4, individuals value laws and rules which they attempt to uphold, and consider it right that they should contribute to society in a positive way. During Stage 4 there is a definite shift away from the interpersonal, towards the societal.

Kohlberg's final level, 'postconventional morality', is marked by a continuation of conformity to laws and rules, if they are for the common good of all, and by the further development of personal values and morals. Whilst at Level 2, individuals see authority as being external to themselves, at Level 3, individuals will see themselves as part of authority, or at least in a position to influence authority. Postconventional morality consumes two stages, although it is doubtful as to whether many individuals ever move beyond Level 2. During Stage 5, individuals continue to acknowledge rules and laws as being important in terms of the maintenance of order. However, they may question those laws and rules as being wrong or unfair. During Stage 6, moral development is characterized by thinking and acting according to universal and self-chosen ethical principles, even if those principles conflict with existing societal laws and rules. At Stage 6, individuals will fight to change societal rules, if they believe them to be wrong. This final stage is rarely reached by individuals.

The application of Kohlberg's work to adolescent behaviour is interesting and offers some explanation of adolescent behaviour (see Chapter 9). Rest (1986) suggests that in early adolescence it is rare to find individuals who have reached the stage of conventional morality, but that in middle adolescence Stages 3 and 4 can be observed. Most adults continue to reason at these stages. There is evidence to suggest, however, that moral development does vary from culture to culture (Snarey *et al.* 1985), and that there are gender differences (Gilligan 1982) possibly associated with gender rules learned in childhood.

Peer relationships

Peer relationships become increasingly important during adolescence and peers, to a certain extent, take over from the family in relation to some aspects of psychosocial functioning. That is not to say that the family becomes any less important, but that adolescents begin to interact with family in a different and more independent way (see Chapter 2). The previous dependence upon family, observed during childhood, is not transferred to peers, although some adolescents do form intense peer relationships which can be described as dependent. It is however more usual for peers to provide a mechanism of support, and a reference group with which the adolescent can begin to identify. One 13 year old girl described the role of friends and how friends differ in their function from the family:

> 'Friends are great to shop with and have a laugh with. They help you with stuff and give you truthful answers. You can tell them things and share things with them, share secrets. You can go to "friend" things with friends and we cheer each other up. You love friends in a "friend" way. You spend a lot of time with family, you live with them permanently, eat with them and talk about school etc. Families take *you* out. They are good for getting money from. You love them in a *family* way.'

This transition from almost total dependence upon family during childhood to the reciprocal relationship with friends is an interesting one. As strong family ties weaken, ties are formed with same-sex peers, and are then partially replaced by ties with opposite-sex peers. This partial and continuous replacement of ties is characterized by increased independence, a growing cognitive awareness and the development of moral reasoning.

The view of the adolescent leaving the secure and comfortable family nest and striving towards a comfortable nest with an opposite-sex partner, is of course a stereotypical example which has little bearing on the lives of many adolescents. In reality the pathway from adolescence to adulthood rarely runs so smoothly. First of all, we can not assume that all children enter the process of adolescence with an equal degree of dependence upon the family. Secondly, the formation of peer relationships is complex and, in identifying with peers, conflict within the family can occur. Finally, we should not assume that all adolescents do engage successfully in peer relationships, or that they are ultimately striving towards a secure relationship with an opposite-sex peer.

Patterns of peers group interaction

As adolescents develop physically and psychologically, the structure of peer groups change. In some early research, Dunphy (1963) showed that initially same-sex peer groups are the norm, but eventually small peer groups combine to form heterosexual 'crowds'. These crowds allow the adolescent to mix socially with members of the opposite sex, and eventually couples will pair off (although it should not be assumed that all pairing off will be heterosexual). Later research by Blyth *et al.* (1982) suggest that patterns of peer interaction remain similar with the percentage of opposite-sex friends increasing with age. Same-sex peers remain important throughout adolescence. By late adolescence, though, while friends remain close, characteristically they allow each other more space and independence.

Gender differences in the formation of relationships

We have already discussed the differences between male and female adolescents in terms of their physiological and psychological development. Gender differences also exist in relation to the development of peer relationships, although the extent to which these differences result from different rates of physical and psychological development is unknown. Certainly, girls tend to form opposite sex relationships and join heterosexual crowds at an earlier age than boys, probably because of their more advanced physical development. The number of friends and the intensity of friendships also appear to vary according to gender. Rutter (1979) suggests that same-sex friendships among male adolescents tend to be much wider, and will include more individuals whereas girls tend to have more intense friendships with fewer individuals. This view is, in part, in contrast to the views of others (see Conger 1991) who consider that girls have more numerous friendships than do boys.

Peer group conformity

We have already suggested that peers become important during adolescence particularly because they provide a reference group from which the adolescent can draw guidance about personal intentions and behaviour. Peer influence, however, is not always positive, and there can be pressure upon the individual to conform to the norms and values of the peer group, even if those norms and values conflict with those held by the individual. Parry-Jones (1985) suggests that for the majority of adolescents, parental influence remains strong. However levels of delinquency and antisocial behaviour suggest that this is not always so. It is important to recognize that not all parents influence their children in a positive way and that, for certain individuals, the peer group may override parents. From the earlier discussion relating to the development of morality, we discussed how in early adolescence most individuals will be reasoning at the preconventional level, and will tend to conform to those who are physically more powerful than they are. For some adolescents, the peer group may be perceived as being more powerful and the adolescent is therefore more likely to conform to them, although Botvin (1984) suggests that self-esteem, self-confidence and personal autonomy are important factors in minimizing conformity to peer pressure.

For adolescents who do conform to peer pressure and engage in negative behaviour, but do not hold personal beliefs and values consistent with the behaviour, internal conflict can arise. This conflict between behaviour and beliefs, known as 'cognitive dissonance', was first described by Festinger (1957) and has greatly influenced research in social psychology. He hypothesized that individuals wish to avoid inconsistency in terms of what they believe and how they behave. In order to resolve conflict the individual has two fundamental choices:

- to change behaviour to conform with personal beliefs;
- to change beliefs to conform with behaviour.

For some adolescents the first option may present difficulties. We have already discussed the strong desire that adolescents have to belong, and not belonging or fear of not belonging can strongly influence behaviour. The lonely adolescent, who desperately wants to belong to a peer group, may well conform to the group's practices just to feel a sense of belonging. For example, Pallikkathayil and Tweed (1983) describe how adolescent drug abusers often begin taking drugs because they want to associate with a peer group (see Chapter 9). Resolving dissonance by stopping drug abuse would probably mean alienation from the peer group, and a return to the loneliness which the adolescent has probably experienced before and dreads feeling again.

The implications for nurses

This chapter has focused upon several theories which make postulations about the nature of psychological development during adolescence. Clearly adolescents develop in a number of domains but the developmental process will vary within each individual and between domains. Adolescents become more independent and will become more capable of making informed choices and decisions. However, the rate at which they develop such skills will vary between individuals and is subject to a number of extraneous variables. It is therefore important that nurses who are working with adolescents recognize individual differences in development because of the need to ensure that communication and interaction with individuals is both appropriate and pertinent. It is only by careful assessment that nurses can begin to understand the complex nature of individuals and of adolescents as a group.

References

Adams, B. (1983) Adolescent health care: needs, priorities and services. *The Nursing Clinics of North America*, 18(2): 237–248.

Agras, W.S. and Kirkley, B.G. (1986) Bulimia: theories of aetiology. In: *Handbook of Eating Disorders*. (Eds K.D. Brownell and J.P. Foreyt). Basic Books, New York.

Blyth, D., Hill, J. and Thiel, K. (1982) Early adolescents significant others: grade and gender differences in perceived relationship with familial and non-familial adults and young people. *Journal of Adolescence and Youth*, 11, 425–440.

Botvin, G. (1984) The Life Skills Training Model: a broad spectrum approach to the prevention of cigarette smoking. In: *Health Education and Youth*. (Ed. G. Campbell). Falmer Press, London.

Buskist, W. and Gerbing, D.W. (1990) *Psychology: Boundaries and Frontiers.* Scott Foresman/Little, Brown, Illinois.

Conger, J.J. (1991) *Adolescence and Youth*, 4th edn. Harper Collins, New York.

Dunphy, D.C. (1963) The social structure of urban adolescent peer groups. *Sociometry*, 26, 230–246.

Erikson, E.H. (1965) *Childhood and Society*. Penguin Books, Harmondsworth.

Festinger, L. (1957) *A Theory of Cognitive Dissonance*. Stanford University Press, Stanford.

Gilligan, C. (1982) *In a Different Voice: Psychological Theory and Women's Development*. Harvard University Press, Cambridge, Mass.

Graham, P. and Rutter, M. (1985) Adolescent disorders. In: *Child and Adolescent Psychiatry*, 2nd edn. (Eds M. Rutter and L. Hersov). Blackwell Scientific Publications, Oxford.

Livson, N. and Peskin, H. (1982) Perspectives in adolescence from longitudinal research. In: *Handbook of Adolescent Psychology*. (Ed. J. Adelson). John Wiley, Chichester.

Marcia, J.E. (1982) Identity in adolescence. In: *Handbook of Adolescent Psychology*. John Wiley, Chichester.

Mussen, P.H., Conger, J.J., Kagan, J. and Huston, A.C. (1990) *Child Development and Personality*, 7th edn. Harper and Row, New York.

Pallikkathayil, L. and Tweed, S. (1983) Substance abuse: alcohol and drugs during adolescence. *Nursing Clinics of North America*, 18(2): 313–321.

Parry-Jones, W.Ll. (1985) Adolescent disturbance. In: *Child and Adolescent Psychiatry*, 2nd edn. (Eds. M. Rutter and L. Hersov). Blackwell Scientific Publications, Oxford.

Petersen, A.C. (1987) The nature of biological–psychosocial interactions: the sample case of early adolescence. In: *Biological– Psychosocial Interactions in Early Adolescence*. (Eds R.M. Lerner and T.T. Foch). Lawrence Erlbaum Associates, New Jersey.

Piaget, J. (1952) *The Origins of Intelligence in Children*. International Universities Press, New York.

Rest, J.R. (1986) *Moral Development: Advances in Research and Theory*. Praeger, New York.

Rutter, M. (1979) *Changing Youth in a Changing Society*. The Nuffield Provincial Hospitals Trust, London.

Snarey, J.R., Reimer, J. and Kohlberg, L. (1985) Development of social–moral reasoning among Kibbutz adolescents: a longitudinal cross-sectional study. *Developmental Psychology*, 21, 3–17.

Tobias, A.L. and Gordan, J.B. (1980) Social consequences of obesity *Journal of The American Dietetic Association*, 76, 338–342.

Tobin-Richards, M., Boxer, A. and Petersen, A.C. (1984) The psychological impact of pubertal change: sex differences in perceptions of self during early adolescence. In: *Girls at Puberty: Biological, Psychological and Social Perspectives*. (Eds J. Brooks-Gunn and A.C. Petersen). Plenum Press, New York.

Vaughan, V.C. and Litt, I.F. (1990) *Child and Adolescent Development: Clinical Implications*. W.B. Saunders, Philadelphia.

Further reading

Rutter, M. and Hersov, L. (eds) (1985) *Child and Adolescent Psychiatry*, 2nd edn. Blackwell Scientific Publications, Oxford.
    This excellent tome contains several chapters exploring factors which influence development throughout childhood and adolescence. Chapters 3 and 21 provide particularly good reviews of work undertaken in this field.

Vaughan, V.C. and Litt, I.F. (1990) *Child and Adolescent Development: Clinical Implications.* W.B. Saunders, Philadelphia.
This book provides a good account of variations in development. The sections on physical development are especially pertinent.

Chapter 4
The Developmental Tasks of Adolescence

In the first three chapters of this book we have focused on the nature of adolescence, the influence of family and friends, and individual differences in development. These discussions have, we hope, provided the foundation for understanding what adolescence is, and those factors which may influence the development of individual adolescents or groups of adolescents. What we have not done, so far, is to clarify in any detail what the process of adolescence entails and it is to this that we now turn our attention.

Typically, the literature refers to the developmental 'tasks' of adolescence (McKinney *et al.* 1977; Rogers 1980; Adams 1983). These tasks provide a much needed structure for analysing the nature of the psychosocial development which occurs between childhood and adulthood. The developmental tasks, according to Conger (1991), must be mastered if the adolescent is to function effectively in adult society. Whilst we agree with Conger that the process of adolescence involves meeting new challenges and achieving a guiding set of norms and beliefs which can provide a framework of adult living, we have some difficulty with the notion of 'mastering' psychosocial tasks. This idea suggests that developmental tasks are rather like a series of tests which you can pass or fail (such as a driving test for example). If you pass, you are considered competent for life in that task and will probably never have to take that particular test again. Psychosocial development, however, is much more complex than driving a car and to suggest that individuals ever reach competence in all (or indeed any) of the developmental tasks is unrealistic. It is more useful to view the developmental tasks in terms of several continuum along which adolescents (and adults) can move *in either direction*, although you would clearly expect adolescents to make some forward progress during the period of time between childhood and adulthood. With this view in mind we will, in this chapter, explore the developmental tasks of adolescence which will enable nurses to have a greater understanding of psychosocial development which in turn may provide a useful basis for examining the potential effects of ill health during adolescence.

The developmental tasks we have chosen to explore are based loosely on the work of McKinney *et al.* (1977). They do not comprise a complete list, but are those tasks which we feel are most pertinent in this context. They are:

- adjusting to a rapidly changing physique and sexual development;
- achieving a sense of independence from parents;
- acquiring the social skills of a young adult;
- developing necessary academic and vocational skills;
- achieving a sense of oneself as a worthwhile person; and
- developing an internalized set of guiding norms and values.

Adjusting to a rapidly changing physique and sexual development

Changing physique and body image

In Chapter 3 we discuss the physiological changes which occur during adolescence and the impact of early and late physical maturation. Adolescents have little control over their physiological maturation and need to ultimately adjust and accept the changes that occur to their bodies. There is, however, evidence to suggest that adolescents, particularly females, are at great risk of developing preoccupations with body image (Cash *et al.* (1986). Girls experience the physical changes which occur at puberty in a more negative way than do boys (Gavin and Furman 1989). This preoccupation with body shape and weight may ultimately result in problems such as anorexia nervosa and bulimia (see Chapter 7).

Why some adolescent girls develop eating disorders in which they exhibit a fear of normal weight is largely unknown (Gowers *et al.* 1991) but is potentially due to culturally defined messages portrayed by the media about the 'ideal' body shape and weight. Dietz (1990) suggests that cultural messages associated with obesity tend to be internalized during adolescence, resulting in 'body ideals' which are often impossibly thin. This point was emphasized by Hill *et al.* (1992) in a study of girls attending an independent school in the north of England. They found that the ideal body shape described by their subjects was significantly slimmer than their current body shape. A disturbing aspect of this particular study is that even girls who were considered to be underweight had felt motivated to diet, leading Hill and colleagues to conclude that actual body weight and weight index had little to do with feelings about dieting. Even those girls who did not need to diet felt they should. These findings are supported by Moses *et al.* (1989) who found that 70% of the girls they studied had dieted in order to lose weight.

It is not difficult therefore to see that if adolescents who do not have major problems with their actual body shape are obsessed with their body image, then adolescents who experience illness or disability which does affect their physical appearance are likely to be even more affected. There is ample evidence to suggest that this is the case. For example, Engstrom (1992) found, in a study of adolescents with inflammatory bowel disease, that they appear to have significantly lower body images than do healthy controls. Adolescents with cancer who face hair loss are also likely to experience decreased body images (Lansdown and Goldman 1988). Similarly, adolescents with severe burns are likely to experience such problems (Favaloro 1988), as are adolescents with skeletal dysfunction such as scoliosis (Jackson 1988).

Sexual development

Sexual development is also an area which may cause concern to some young people and may be linked to body image. Gowers *et al.* (1991), for example, found that pre-pubescent anorectic girls exhibited anxiety in relation to their impending menarche as well as a fear of obesity. There are also a number of psychosexual disorders which are prominent during adolescence and which may cause extreme anxiety to afflicted individuals (see Zucker and Green 1992 for a review). Adolescents who have been sexually abused as children or during adolescence may be in particular need of counselling in relation to psychosexual disorder. Watkins and Bentovim (1992) suggest that these young people are likely to be particularly confused about their emerging sexuality and sexual identity.

A further group of young people who we should consider are those who have to make choices about their future sexual behaviour because of the fear of transmitting illness onto their own children. For example, adolescents with sickle cell anaemia, thalassaemia, haemophilia and cystic fibrosis have to make important decisions in relation to their own relationships and the possible impact that their illness may have on any children they may one day have. The possibility that their children may inherit their own faulty genes can cause great distress and anxiety (Taylor 1994). Additionally, some adolescents have to live with the knowledge that they themselves are unlikely to live to see their own children growing up. These anxieties become very real to young people, particularly when they meet potential sexual partners. There is clearly a need at this stage, if not before, for skilled genetic counselling in order to help the young people involved to be knowledgeable about potential risks.

Adolescents, then, are particularly prone to anxiety over body image and emerging sexuality. These anxieties may become magnified when young people have an illness or disability, particularly if that illness or disability affects outward appearance or carries the potential for genetic transmission. Such young people require sensitive care but it should be acknowledged that reactions will depend upon such variables as the nature of the condition, family support, the reaction of peers and the personality of the adolescent involved. Enabling the adolescent outwardly to express anxiety is useful and referring adolescents, where appropriate, to the genetic counselling services is important. There is also a great deal that nurses can do to help adolescents come to terms with body image and emerging sexuality. Nurses in school, for example, can help young people to explore the role of the media in the formation of their ideal body images and facilitate discussion which can dispel some of the myths regarding the supposed correlation between happiness and thinness.

Achieving a sense of independence from parents

As we discuss in some depth in Chapter 2, achieving a sense of independence from parents is an important feature of adolescence. Young people strive to loosen the previously held ties and control held by parents in order to develop their own sense of identity (Erikson 1965). This process is affected by a number of variables such as socioeconomic status, culture and particularly health status. There is much evidence which supports the fact that illness and disability may severely affect the adolescent's ability to find and maintain independence.

Gaining independence is not, however, a one way process. Parents too, as adolescents develop, will usually promote independence and expect adolescents to take some degree of responsibility for their own health status (Susman *et al.* 1992). Unfortunately, this promotion of independence is less evident in parents of ill and disabled young people. In an early study by Anderson and Clarke (1982), adolescents with cerebral palsy and spina bifida were less likely to be afforded the same degree of independence as were unaffected adolescents. Gillies (1992) also found that parents were reluctant to afford independence to chronically ill adolescents. Of the 30% of adolescents studied who required special care at home, only 5% of mothers enabled adolescents to cope independently.

Dependence on parents may however be a necessity and the subtle differences between parents who have to keep adolescents relatively dependent upon them and those who choose to do so should be acknowledged by nurses. Adolescents with cystic fibrosis, for example, may be physically dependent on their parents for physiotherapy (Simmons *et al.* 1985) whereas other parents, for a variety of reasons, may deny adolescents independence even when it is reasonable that they could become self-caring. Conflict may arise as a result of the adolescents' need for independence and the parents' need for control (Susman *et al.* 1993) and nurses can, if they are not careful, find themselves in the middle of a controlling parent and a frustrated adolescent. Nurses can however do a great deal to diffuse the situation. Parents should be helped to realize that although adolescents may be dependent for some aspects of their physical care, they have a need to be granted a degree of emotional freedom. Even in relation to physical care, it is possible for some adolescents to be taught skills which will give them more independence. Dryden (1989), for example, suggests that adolescents can be taught practical skills such as passing nasogastric tubes which enable them a greater degree of independence.

Dying adolescents are a group who we feel are particularly vulnerable in terms of gaining independence particularly if the adolescent is in hospital. Hospitalization itself runs the risk of infanticizing adolescents (Gillies, 1992), but when the adolescent is dying this problem can be magnified. It is important for nurses to realize that the dying adolescent probably has a normal desire for independence (Papadatou 1989), even though their condition may prevent them from achieving it. Careful assessment and planning of care, and ensuring that adolescents are included in decision making can help to overcome some of their feelings of inadequacy and frustration. Simple concessions such as allowing adolescents to stay up late, or make a cup of tea in the ward kitchen are measures which reduce dependence and are hardly likely to put any strain on stretched health service resources.

Achieving the social skills of an adult

The social skills of adulthood will clearly vary from culture to culture and adolescents learn what those skills are through a variety of sources including the family, the education system, the media and their peers. The process of learning these skills is not something that begins or ends with adolescence, but has its origins in early childhood (see Chapter 2) and continues long into adulthood. There are few of us, when faced with a new situation during our adult years, who do not experience some anxiety about how we should behave or what social skills are required.

The task of achieving the social skills of an adult is clearly linked with the process of gaining independence from parents and again we find that adolescents with illness or disability may experience problems. For example, young people with disabilities were found by Anderson and Clarke (1982) to be severely restricted in their social interaction outside of the family context which minimized their social experiences. It is important however that young people do interact with their peers and other adults so that their choice of role models for adult behaviour is not limited. This is particularly important where parents do not provide good role models in terms of social skills. Eiser (1990) suggests that the holiday clubs which have been commonplace in the USA for a number of years may be useful in enabling young people to mix with other adults and peers in an environment away from parents but which has medical and nursing help on hand if required. Such camps may provide a variance in role models for those adolescents who lead somewhat restricted lives (see Chapter 2).

There is also evidence to suggest that adolescents worry about exhibiting adult social skills rather than childish ones when they are unwell. Favaloro (1988), in her study of adolescents with burn injuries, found that adolescents had particular difficulties in relation to the expression of pain. Some of the adolescents held the belief that expression of pain is not socially acceptable in adulthood and therefore denied its existence. Favaloro suggests that adolescents need to be helped to find mature emotional control in these instances which requires a great deal of skill and understanding on the part of the nurses. It is perhaps a fault of our society that we, as adults, do not readily show emotion in public, and so adolescents have little chance of learning appropriate emotional responses. This is particularly relevant when adolescents are in hospital and have little opportunity for privacy.

Developing academic and vocational skills

Choosing employment, and developing the necessary academic and vocational skills, are important features of adolescence. From early childhood adults ask, 'What do you want to be when you grow up?' Children usually reply by naming a vocation which may or may not be feasible. During adolescence, young people have to make serious decisions about their future role in society. From the age of 13 or 14, decisions about examination options are made, and it is difficult if not impossible to make vast changes once a particular course has been set.

For some young people, however, the choice is not between which

GCSE they should take, but rather whether they will be able to get a job at all when they leave school. Cairns *et al.* (1991) in a study in Northern Ireland found that high unemployment in the area was a source of great stress to adolescents. Rutter (1989) suggests that the effectiveness of the school contributes towards the employment status of the individual after school. Less effective schools had poor attendance records, poor attenders tended to leave school early with a lack of scholastic qualifications and enter either unskilled employment or have a very poor employment record. This is perhaps rather a simplistic view and Rutter does not explore adequately what he defines as 'effective'. Schools tend to be products of the social environment as well as contributing towards it.

Adolescents with ill health or disability can face a difficult task when deciding about their future choices. Some choices are unfortunately limited by physical condition. For example, adolescents with juvenile rheumatoid arthritis, and deaf adolescents may find that some career avenues are closed to them (Beales *et al.* 1983; Cole and Edelman 1991) which can be the source of distress.

Illness and disability, which involves periods of long or frequent hospitalization, can also clearly have an impact on schooling and/or work. Whilst in hospital it is important that adolescents who are still at school are allowed to continue with their studies. They may need assistance from the hospital teacher, although it may be more appropriate to contact the school and request that specific work be sent in. A Save the Children Fund survey (1989) found that almost half of hospital teachers have a background in early years teaching and may not feel comfortable teaching older patients. With older adolescents who are working on specific course work, a quiet place to study may be more appropriate than enforcing attendance at a mixed age hospital school. Research into the effect of chronic illness and disability on school performance has shown varying results and probably is dependent upon factors such as hospitalization, as well as the age of diagnosis, the nature of treatment, the natural course of the illness and the family situation (see Eiser 1990, for a review).

Our final area of discussion in this section relates to dying adolescents who can experience particular difficulties in relation to this task, as can the nurses who are caring for them. Papadatou (1989) suggests that even though the adolescent is dying it is important to give meaning and purpose to life in order to help the young person cope with the reality of the situation. These individuals need to 'discard their unfulfilled dreams, expectations and goals' but should be encouraged to talk about them as part of the discarding process. It is important to remember that dying adolescents may go through a grieving process as they accept the loss of their future. Encouraging expression of feeling can be cathartic and avoid feelings of social isolation. Focusing on very short term goals, whilst they are not the same, can bring some optimism to their lives (Papadatou 1989).

Achieving a sense of oneself as a worthwhile person

Developing a sense of self-worth is an important part of adolescence and involves evaluating one's own qualities and activities. Many adolescents hold very strong ideological views and are perturbed by some elements of their social world. They may try to alter what they perceive to be adverse features of their worlds and such activities can contribute to feelings of self-worth. The concept of self-worth is strongly linked to the notion of *self-esteem* which, according to Rosenberg (1985), involves making judgements about our own competences in relation to our own internal standards. We describe young people as having high or low self-esteem depending upon the extent to which they feel they are living up to their own internalized values.

Adolescents who are ill or disabled may find it difficult to develop a sense of self-worth because of the limitations placed upon them by their illness, and because they may perceive themselves to be a burden on their carers (Muller *et al.* 1992). Midence *et al.* (1993), for example, suggest that adolescents with sickle cell anaemia may have low self-esteem, particularly if they experience frequent sickle cell crises and require frequent hospitalization. Favaloro (1988) also noted that adolescents with burns in hospital may have low self-esteem and feelings of reduced self-worth.

Nurses can help young people to develop a greater sense of self-worth by involving them in decisions and discussions about their own care and by promoting self-care. It may also be useful to explore with adolescents their own feelings of deficit in relation to social or political activities they would like to become involved in. It may be that, whilst they cannot play the role they would like, they can be involved in other related activities.

Developing an internalized set of norms and values

This final task of adolescence is closely linked to self-worth and self-esteem and refers to being able to make one's own decisions about issues. It is part of the socialization process of acquiring attitudes and values which are compatible with society's. Adolescents may question the norms and values of those around them even though they have accepted those norms and values previously. Their growing cognitive ability and awareness allows them to see beyond the 'here and now' and to use deductive reasoning to think beyond the immediate consequences of their own actions and those of others.

Nurses involved with adolescents should try to ensure that they do not limit the development of norms and values, particularly when adolescents are in hospital, which typically impose their own norms and values on the people they care for (Muller *et al.* 1992). We pick this point up in the next section.

The implications for nurses

Clearly the developmental tasks of adolescence which we have chosen to highlight overlap with each other a great deal. The process of gaining independence from parents, for example, is pivotal to the achievement of other tasks, and the last two tasks we have discussed interrelate to a large extent. Thus whilst we have separated the tasks for the purposes of this discussion, it is important to recognize the integrative nature of the developmental process.

Nurses who are involved with the care of adolescents can play an important role in facilitating young people in relation to developmental tasks (Mackenzie 1988; Gillies 1992). In Chapter 6, we discuss aspects of hospital services for adolescents, and clearly hospitals can do a great deal to help or limit psychosocial development. As we have discussed there are already potential difficulties for adolescents with ill health or disability in terms of the development or achievement of tasks and we would like to believe that hospitalization does not make the situation any worse. In the absence of specific adolescent units we would urge paediatric and adult units which provide care for adolescents to re-appraise their policies and adhere to the guidance proffered by Action for Sick Children (1990), the Department of Health (1991) and the Audit Commission (1993) (see Chapter 6).

Finally, in terms of the individualized care that nurses deliver we suggest a number of simple measures which can help adolescents when they are in hospital. First, nurses can do much to ensure that the environment is suitable for adolescents. The provision of somewhere quiet to study, bathrooms which the adolescents can lock, allowing access to beverages, and being flexible about 'lights out' times, are all examples of simple measures which can make all the difference to the adolescent. Clearly where there is the potential for disturbing other patients, rules should be negotiated and boundaries established. Second, nurses can ensure that they involve adolescents in decision making and care planning and promote self-care wherever it is feasible. This may also involve helping parents to come to terms with the fact that, even though their children are ill, they need to have control over their own lives and to be as independent as possible. This is more difficult for some parents than for others and allowing parents to talk through their fears can help to resolve areas of conflict and concern. Third, nurses can help adolescents to become comfortable with their own bodies, particularly if their illness (or treatment) results in changes to their physical appearance. Adolescents with cancer who may lose their hair, or who have to undergo mutilating surgery, need particular care (Thompson 1990), as do those with skeletal problems such as scoliosis (Jackson, 1988) or with burn injuries (Favaloro 1988).

Finally, adolescence is a period during which young people make choices about their future roles as adults, and come to develop a sense of being a worthwhile member of society. Ensuring that educational aspirations are facilitated rather than hampered by hospitalization and ill health is an important part of providing effective care. Where the potential for choice of vocation is limited by illness or impending death, nurses can be of great assistance in allowing the young person time to express feelings of disappointment and frustration.

References

Action for Sick Children (1990) *Setting Standards for Adolescents in Hospital.* NAWCH Quality Review Series. ACS, London.

Adams, B.N. (1983) Adolescent health care: needs, priorities and services. *Nursing Clinics of North America*, 18(2): 237–248.

Anderson, E.M. and Clarke, L. (1982) *Disability in Adolescence.* Methuen, London.

Audit Commission (1993) *Children First: A Study of Hospital Services.* HMSO, London.

Beales, J.G., Keen, J.H. and Lennox-Holt, P.J. (1983) The child's perception of the disease and the experience of pain in juvenile chronic arthritis. *Journal of Rheumatology*, 10: 61–65.

Cairns, E., McWhirter, L., Barry, R. and Duffy, U. (1991) The development of well-being in late adolescence. *Journal of Child Psychology and Psychiatry*, 32(4): 635–643.

Cash, T.F., Winstead, B.A. and Janda, L.H. (1986) Body image survey report: the great American shape-up. *Psychology Today*, 20: 30–37.

Cole, S.H. and Edelman, R.J. (1991) Identity patterns and self-and teacher-perceptions of problems for deaf adolescents: a research note. *Journal of Child Psychology and Psychiatry*, 32(7): 1159–1165.

Conger, J.J. (1991) *Adolescence and Youth*, 4th edn. Harper Collins, New York.

Department of Health (1991) *Welfare of Children and Young People in Hospital.* HMSO, London.

Dietz, W.H. (1990) You are what you eat – what you eat is what you are. *Journal of Adolescent Health Care,* 11: 76–81.

Dryden, S. (1989) Paediatric medicine in the community. *Paediatric Nursing,* 1(8): 17–18.

Eiser, C. (1990) Psychological effects of chronic disease. *Journal of Child Psychology and Psychiatry,* 31(1): 85–98.

Engstrom, I. (1992) Mental health and psychological functioning in children and adolescents with inflammatory bowel disease: a comparison with children having other chronic illnesses and with healthy children. *Journal of Child Psychology and Psychiatry,* 33(3): 563–582.

Erikson, E. (1965) *Childhood and Society.* Penguin, Harmondsworth.

Favaloro, R. (1988) Adolescent development and implications for pain management. *Pediatric Nursing,* 14(1): 27–29.

Gavin, L.A. and Furman, W. (1989) Age difference in adolescents' perceptions of their peer groups. *Developmental Psychology,* 25: 827–834.

Gillies, M. (1992) Teenage traumas. *Nursing Times,* 88(27): 26–29.

Gowers, S.G., Crisp, A.H., Joughin, N. and Bhat, A. (1991) Premenarcheal anorexia nervosa. *Journal of Child Psychology and Psychiatry,* 32(3): 515–524.

Hill, A.J., Oliver, S. and Rogers, P.J. (1992) Eating in the adult world: the rise of dieting in childhood and adolescence. *British Journal of Clinical Psychology,* 31: 95–105.

Jackson, R. (1988) Scoliosis in juvenile and adolescent children. *Health Visitor,* 61: 76–77.

Lansdown, R. and Goldman, A. (1988) The psychological care of children with malignant disease. *Journal of Child Psychology and Psychiatry,* 29(5): 555–568.

Mackenzie, H. (1988) Teenagers in hospital. *Nursing Times,* 84(32): 58–61.

McKinney, J.P., Fitzgerald, H.E. and Strommen, E.A. (1977) *The Adolescent and Young Adult.* Dorsey Press, Illinois.

Midence, K., Fuggle, P. and Davies, S.C. (1993) Psychological aspects of sickle cell disease (SCD) in childhood and adolescence: a review. *British Journal of Clinical Psychology,* 32: 271–280.

Moses, N., Banilivy, M.M. and Lifshitz, F. (1989) Fear of obesity among adolescent girls. *Pediatrics,* 93: 393–398.

Muller, D.J., Harris, P.J., Wattley, L. and Taylor, J. (1992) *Nursing Children: Psychology, Research and Practice,* 2nd edn. Chapman and Hall, London.

Papadatou, D. (1989) Caring for dying adolescents. *Nursing Times,* 85(18): 28–31.

Rogers, D. (1980) *Adolescents and Youth.* Prentice Hall, Englewood Cliffs, New Jersey.

Rosenberg, M. (1985) Self-concept and psychological well being in adolescence. In: *The Development of Self.* (Ed. R.L. Heahy). Academic Press, Orlando, Florida.

Rutter, M. (1989) Pathways from childhood to adult life. *Journal of Child Psychology and Psychiatry,* 30(1): 23–51.

Save the Children Fund (1989) Play provision in hospital. *Paediatric Nursing,* 1(3): 19–20.

Simmons, R.J., Corey, M., Cowen, L., Kennan, N., Robertson, J. and Levison, H. (1985) Emotional adjustments of early adolescents with cystic fibrosis. *Psychosomatic Medicines,* 47(2): 111–121.

Susman, E.J., Dorn, L.D., Feagans, L.V. and Ray, W.J. (1992) Historical and theoretical perspectives on behavioral health in children and adolescents: an introduction. In: *Emotion, Cognition, Health and Development in Children and Adolescents.* (Eds E.J. Susman, L.V. Feagans and W.J. Ray). Lawrence Erlbaum Associates, Hillsdale, New Jersey.

Taylor, J. (1994) The sick and well adolescent. In: *Health Promotion and Patient Education.* (Ed. P. Webb). Chapman and Hall, London.

Thompson, J. (1990) The adolescent with cancer. In: *The Child with Cancer.* (Ed. J. Thompson). Scutari Press, London.

Watkins, B. and Bentovim, A. (1992) The sexual abuse of male children and adolescents: a review of current research. *Journal of Child Psychology and Psychiatry,* 33(1): 197–248.

Zucker, K.J. and Green, R. (1992) Psychosexual disorders in children and adolescents. *Journal of Child Psychology and Psychiatry,* 33(1): 107–151.

Further reading

Rutter, M. (1989) Pathways from childhood to adult life. *Journal of Child Psychology and Psychiatry,* 30(1): 23–51.

This excellent paper reviews principles and concepts of development giving consideration to development in its social context, the timing of experiences, parallels and differences between normal and abnormal development, key life transitions, and risk and protective factors. It provides a particularly good review of longitudinal studies in this field.

Chapter 5
Health Promotion

Health promotion strategies and the making of healthy choices can, in some instances, have life-long effects in terms of both physiological, and psychosocial health. Nurses working in a variety of settings will have opportunities, both formal and informal, to impart information to adolescents and their families about health and healthy living. However, in order to be effective health promoters in the field of adolescent health, nurses need to ensure that the way in which they promote health is appropriate and relevant. An understanding of the social contexts in which adolescents function, cognisance of the way in which adolescents learn and the influences upon that learning is essential. This chapter will explore strategies for maximizing the effectiveness of health promotion, by focusing on the ways in which adolescents learn and understand.

Learning

The way in which humans learn has been the focus of much speculation over the last century or so. Early psychologists tended to be aligned to one of two schools of thought. One school held to the theory that behaviour, and thereby learning, was innate and that most behaviour occurred as a result of instinct. In other words that behaviour is genetically determined. William McDougall (1871–1938) was a principal psychologist who held such a view (see Burkist and Gerbing 1990). The second school of thought, led by John Watson (1878–1958), held that most behaviour, and thereby learning, results through interaction with the environment. Modern psychologists tend not to align themselves forcefully to either school, but acknowledge that learning probably results from a combination of both genetic and environmental influence. As human beings we are genetically programmed to be able to learn through interaction with the environment, and our behaviour will be modified according to environmental influence.

The two most important theories of learning when considering adolescent learning and health promotions are those proposed by Thorndike (1874–1949) and later by Skinner (1904–1990) (see Burkist and Gerbing 1990). A further theory, based on Skinner's work and then further elaborated and defined, was proposed by Bandura (1977). Thorndike's work was very much involved with the study of animal behaviour. Skinner's work on operant conditioning, however, is of interest in the study of human behaviour as he postulated that behaviour could, and would, be influenced by its consequences. Thus humans are influenced by the effects of their behaviour, and will modify future behaviour in light of the effect of previous behaviour. For example, an adolescent who gets 'grounded' after staying out beyond a deadline may think twice before breaking the deadline a second time. The adolescent's behaviour may change and he or she is more likely to stick to house rules in future because of the detrimental consequences of breaking those rules. The punishment received as a result of behaviour is said to weaken similar future behaviour patterns. Likewise, if an adolescent takes a younger sibling out to the park and gets extra pocket money for the effort, he or she is more likely to repeat the behaviour in future.

Bandura (1977) expanded on Skinner's theory and further suggested that, whilst behaviour may be affected by its consequences, much of what we learn is through observation of others. We learn behaviour through modelling ourselves on others and through observing the consequences of the behaviour of others. Thus if we observe the behaviour of a friend who gets in trouble at school because of handing in homework late, we learn the consequences of repeating such behaviour ourselves may well be incurring the teacher's displeasure. Bandura proposed that this social learning applies not only to overt behaviours but will also influence our values, beliefs and expectations.

Clearly, the theories of operant conditioning and social learning theory are more complex than suggested above but it is not our intention here to outline them in any depth – for more information see the Further reading section at the end of this chapter. What is important here is the role of learning in relation to health promotion strategies, and a basic understanding of how adolescents learn is fundamental to such strategies. If consideration is given to the complex social worlds of adolescents and the many different people, including peers, the family, teachers and media figures, with whom the adolescent may interact or observe, it perhaps puts the necessity of understanding learning theory into context. The adolescent does not exist within a vacuum but will be basing decisions relating to lifestyle on various influences which include observations as to how particular forms of behaviour are received by others, and through watching the consequences of the behaviour of others, and modifying their behaviour as a result.

Cognitive development

For those involved in health promotion during the period of adolescence, a knowledge of learning theory is of fundamental importance. It is also necessary to have some insight into how adolescents understand their worlds and the information they receive within those worlds. The transition from childhood to adolescence and then to adulthood is marked by development in the way in which information is processed and understood, and consequently in the way in which decisions are made. Jean Piaget (1896–1980) proposed theories which attempted to explain the development of thinking in children and adolescents, and whilst his many works have been the focus of some criticism, chiefly relating to the way in which he undertook his experiments and to the absence of a statistical basis for his work (Beard 1969), the fundamental postulations he made have relevance in the study of adolescents and their understanding.

Piaget believed that the beginning of adolescence marked a new phase of increasing collaboration involving the exchange of viewpoints and discussion of the merits of differing views. This exchange leads to greater mutual understanding and to adolescents placing themselves at points of view which they have not previously held. Consideration of many viewpoints gives the adolescent more flexibility in thinking, and leads to an increasing interest in a variety of social systems. For example, many young people are becoming increasingly aware of the need to conserve the ozone layer because of the environmental effects global warming is having on the southern hemisphere. It also results in adolescents being critical of previously held personal viewpoints. In terms of health promotion strategies, adolescence is a time when previous teaching relating to lifestyle may be questioned and the adolescent comes to realize that what were thought to be unalterable rules and conventions, can indeed be challenged through the process of logical argument.

According to Piagetian theory, the final stage of cognitive development coincides roughly with the onset of adolescence. Piaget called this final stage 'formal operations'. This stage is marked by several discrete changes which are critical to understanding how the adolescent thinks. First of all, the adolescent is able to engage in hypothetico-deductive reasoning. During the preceding stage of concrete operations the child is (usually) unable to focus on the possible, and concentrates on what is real and known. As the child moves into the formal operations period the ability develops to begin to reason in propositions, and to argue by implication. Thus a subtle move in reasoning from the real to the possible is made. The adolescent in the formal operations stage is able to give consideration to a variety of possible consequences. For example, a child may accept that smoking is bad for health and will accept such teaching as true. In formal operations the adolescent will give consideration to the benefits as well as the detriments of smoking, and will form a decision about personal smoking habits after consideration of all potential consequences. The adolescent who has reached the stage of formal operations may also question inconsistencies, such as a school nurse advising of the dangers of smoking, who is then seeing smoking in the staff room, as well as recognizing that there are exceptions to established rules (Botvin 1984) such as, for example, that not all people who smoke get lung cancer.

As well as becoming capable of abstract thinking, the adolescent will also have the capacity to be logical and systematic in decision making. The adolescent learns to solve problems by mentally working through each possible combination to its logical conclusion, eliminating unsupported hypotheses on the way until a successful solution to a problem is found. This second important facet of formal operations also involves adolescents becoming conscious of their own thinking and reflecting upon it in order to provide logical justifications for decision making. Just as adolescents will propose and test hypotheses in order to solve problems in a logical way, so they will also test out their own individual thoughts about a particular topic. Through a process of constantly testing and refining internal values and beliefs, the adolescent should emerge with a set of beliefs which have resulted from a process of refinement and logical thinking.

A further important aspect of adolescents is the way they tend to differ from adults in terms of egocentrism. In the pre-concrete operations stage children are very egocentric, as demonstrated by Piaget in his 'Three Mountains' experiment (see Muller *et al.* 1992). This egocentrism changes slightly during the concrete operations stage and early adolescence but adolescents remain fundamentally egocentric until they are well through the process of adolescence. For example, Conger (1991) suggests that adolescents tend to develop notions that what they are thinking and experiencing is completely new and unique to them and has never been experienced before. Thus when parents, nurses and teachers make remarks such as 'I know exactly how you feel' they will probably be met with a certain amount of scepticism and disbelief.

It is probably true to say however that most of us do not think in abstract terms all the time, and some adults rarely, if ever, are able to think in such terms (Lovell 1961; Keating 1980; Overton *et al.* 1987). Furthermore, there is evidence to suggest that some younger children are capable of formal operational thought. This can cause problems in terms of health promotion as it is not therefore possible to ascertain levels of cognitive thought by having prior knowledge of age (see also Chapter 1). It is true to say that not all adolescents of a given age will have reached the same level of cognitive development, but acknowledging such discrepancies and realizing the need to make individual assessment of cognitive ability is a pre-requisite of a successful health promotion strategy. Tauer (1983) suggests that those who possess knowledge of cognitive domains will undoubtedly be in a better position to offer appropriate education.

Health promotion

The implications of learning theory and theories of cognitive development are vast and raise several questions about how professionals can ensure that health promotion strategies are appropriate. There is no easy answer, particularly as many professionals involved in health promotion are faced with groups of adolescents rather than individuals, which can make it very difficult to assess individual abilities. For example, in a group of 14-year-old adolescents there are likely to be wide variations in ability to comprehend information. If the level of information is too complex some adolescents will become confused and will fail to grasp information. Equally, if information is pitched at a low level, other adolescents will become bored and will 'switch off'.

Models of health promotion

For nurses involved in health promoting activity it is often difficult to define how best they can approach a specific task. Ewles and Simnett (1992) define five models of health promotion which can assist health promoters to define their aims and values. These models are the 'medical approach'; the 'behavioural change approach'; the 'educational approach'; the 'client-centred approach'; and the 'societal change approach'. It is useful for health promoters to decide clearly what the desired outcome of their strategy is, and then to decide which model or combination of models is appropriate to that outcome. The medical approach, for example, aims to prevent medically defined diseases and involves seeking medical intervention in order to remain free of, or become free from, disease or disability. The aim of the health promoter is therefore to promote the value of, for example, immunization against rubella, or of seeking medical assistance if an adolescent suspects they may have contracted a sexually transmitted disease.

The behavioural change approach has a different aim which is to encourage adolescents to change negative health behaviour to positive behaviour. Such an approach would be adopted in relation to teaching a group of adolescents in school about, for example, healthy eating, the value of exercise and not smoking. This approach differs from the educational approach which aims to give the adolescent information as well as ensuring understanding about health behaviour so that they can make an informed approach about lifestyle and health. Ewles and Simnett (1992) suggest that most school health education programmes adopt this approach, which aims to help students acquire the skills for healthy living, as well as knowledge.

The client-centred approach involves working with adolescents on their own terms, helping them to identify their own concerns in relation to health and then facilitating the acquisition of the skills and knowledge to address those concerns. In schools, many nurses are adopting such an approach by running 'surgeries' where adolescents can seek the advice of the school nurse, in privacy, about a wide range of concerns. In these situations it is the adolescent who sets the agenda and the nurse who responds by further empowering adolescents by helping them to seek out information, and facilitating their understanding of information.

The final approach outlined by Ewles and Simnett (1992) is the societal change approach which aims to raise health consciousness at a level beyond the individual, and encourages society to enable individuals to adopt healthier lifestyles and take greater responsibility for their own health. We refer in the next section to the importance of community support in health promoting activities and the societal change approach aims to do just this. For example, there is little point in educating adolescents about the potential dangers of glue sniffing if local shopkeepers continue to make glue and solvents readily available, or of encouraging adolescents to take regular exercise if the local sports facilities are inaccessible to them.

Strategies for effective health promotion

Child (1986) suggests that when introducing new information to adolescents, one should proceed from the concrete to the abstract. Macfarlane and Mcpherson (1992) further suggest that adolescents are far more likely to change negative behaviour if the information they are introduced to relates directly to them as individuals. New concepts should be introduced in an orderly and cumulative fashion so that individuals can internalize concepts in a logical and orderly sequence. The Health Education 13–18 Project (Schools Council/Health Council 1982) also suggests a similar strategy for ensuring that health promotion is effective in meeting the educational needs of adolescents. The principles of their approach involve encouraging individuals to identify with real situations and experiences, that is to say the starting point of any strategy should allow adolescents to think about concrete situations which they have personally experienced. Secondly, adolescents should be encouraged to clarify their own attitudes and values about a particular topic, allowing them to explore and discuss their personal perspective. This second stage focuses again on what the adolescent knows, and allows egocentrism as an acceptable starting point for further discussion. Finally, information should be given in a non-didactic way (Taylor 1994), which allows exchange of views and exploration of options. Thus individuals are encouraged to look at their own practices and current lifestyle in a way which is appropriate to their age, culture and cognitive ability. Each individual is given the opportunity to think about personal experience and already worked through solutions, before giving consideration to alternative viewpoints and new possible solutions.

When handling group situations with adolescents it is also important to recognize the power of group dynamics, and ground rules should be carefully discussed and agreed upon before the opening of discussion. We have already referred to learning theory in the earlier parts of this chapter, and in group learning it is important to acknowledge the potential effects of particular behaviours upon learning within a group. A couple of simple exemplars highlight this point. Take, for example, an adolescent who admits to holding a particular viewpoint which is felt to be controversial by other members of the group. If the individual is made to feel badly about holding such a view, and is ostracized from the rest of the group, he or she is unlikely to be willing to participate in further exchange of views. A fundamental ground rule must be therefore that each individual is entitled to an opinion and should be valued for their viewpoint regardless of how controversial it appears. This is not always as easy to put into practice as it sounds. Take a second examplar, of the adolescent who admits to engaging in antisocial behaviour, such as drug taking. The group could reinforce such behaviour by over focusing interest and attention on the adolescent. Furthermore, other adolescents in the group may observe the somewhat flattering consequences of the deviant behaviour. This negative form of vicarious learning could have potentially serious results. Controlling the reinforcement and punishment of viewpoints within the group situation can then be hazardous and working with such groups should be seen as a skilled activity. A knowledge of members of the group is important, as is background knowledge about current fads and popular media figures. Counter-balancing an adolescent's admission of engaging in deviant behaviour with, for example, reference to media cover of similar deviance can be effective, although care should be taken not to embarrass the deviant individual.

Table 5.1   Some principles of working with adolescents in groups

Do	Don't
Lay down clear ground rules	Break your own ground rules
Involve adolescents	Force participation
Use group discussion	Isolate anyone
Use case studies/role play	Use 'shock horror' tactics
Facilitate sharing of views	Embarrass anyone
Refer to media figures	Get out of date
Start with concrete concepts	Start with abstract concepts

It has not been our intention to be prescriptive here, but rather to suggest that working with groups of adolescents is not always an easy task. To this end we have included in Table 5.1 some important principles of working with adolescents in groups as suggested by Taylor (1994). In addition, Gibson (1987) suggests that health promotion should be effective and action oriented, should be group/activity based, should assume a process rather than a product approach and should use an educational rather than a medical model (see p59–60). There are a great deal of resources and literature available to help those involved in health promotion to plan activities, and lists of material can usually be obtained through local Health Promotion Units. Further information about working with groups is included in the Further reading section at the end of this chapter.

External influences

Working with adolescents in health promotion activities is, as we have already said, a skilled activity which requires knowledge of psychological theory and aptitude in dealing with individuals in group situations. It is also important to give thought to the social world of the adolescent and how that world influences the impact of health promotion.

Throughout childhood various influences impact upon the development of personal value and belief systems. These influences include particularly the family, as well as peers, school, and to a lesser or greater extent, religion and culture (see Chapter 2). French (1984) suggests that these influences should be considered because they provide a filter through which the child and adolescent perceives the outside world and selects and interprets those perceptions. Acknowledgement of the power of these external influences gives support to the view that health promotion should be facilitated by professionals with knowledge of individual adolescents (Taylor 1994). It is also useful, and necessary, to aim health promotion strategies towards external influences as well as at individual adolescents. Kolbe (1984) emphasizes this necessity, and the need to ensure that wider influences allow individuals to change their behaviour, and to reinforce positive behaviour. If health promotion strategies are not widely supported, they are less likely to be effective. Tones *et al.* (1990) suggest that effective health promotion among the young must consider all the potential factors involved in a particular health related behaviour. Seeking the support of family, the local media, shopkeepers and community services is clearly important. For example, if a particular strategy is aimed at reducing smoking among adolescents, engaging the support of shopkeepers to stop them selling cigarettes to young adolescents is of obvious importance, and providing an accessible anti-smoking clinic for adolescent smokers can provide support aimed at helping them to give up. Furthermore, linking such strategies to national campaigns such as National No-Smoking Day can be a successful strategy (Stewart and Orme 1991). The organization of such an approach is clearly far from easy and involves sophisticated levels of networking. It is however worth the effort and the professional involved in health promotion will not be viewed as a lone voice in isolation from other external messages, but will be part of a collaborative programme of education and support. It is also essential when evaluating the effectiveness of any health promotion strategy to look beyond the individual adolescent to the effects upon for example, the school, the family and the wider community (Tones *et al.* 1990).

Levels of prevention

We have already referred to the potentially long lasting effects of negative health behaviour during adolescence. Health promotion encompasses educating individuals, groups and communities about health, but also encompasses the prevention of ill health. Clearly, the rewards of prevention in children and adolescents are great and we now turn to looking at the practical application of preventive programmes which can be influential in the short and longer term health of the adolescent.

Primary prevention

Primary prevention is aimed at healthy individuals and has the intent of preventing ill health. In terms of adolescent health, most health promoting activities undertaken by professionals are primary prevention by nature. For example, immunization during childhood and adolescence is a simple primary prevention activity which aims at preventing the development of infectious disease. Other examples include the promotion of healthy eating which can assist in preventing heart disease during adulthood, and promoting the dangers of smoking in an attempt to prevent respiratory disease and lung cancer.

Primary prevention during adolescence, however, is not a simple activity. We have already referred to the counter-influence which can be involved in changing adolescent behaviour and these influences are also apparent in primary preventive strategies. An example is the promotion of sexual health and the prevention of unwanted pregnancy, cervical carcinoma and sexually transmitted diseases including the human immunodeficiency virus (HIV). The number of adolescents who become sexually active is thought to be high (Curtis *et al.* 1989). Bowie and Ford (1989), in a study of adolescent sexual activity, found that up to 47% of adolescents had engaged in sexual intercourse before the age of 16 years. There is further evidence to suggest that many adolescent girls become pregnant, and many of these will have terminations of pregnancy. The current abortion rate for British adolescent girls is 20.9 per 10 000 (Macfarlane and Mcpherson 1992). Moriasy and Thomas (1990) suggest that, apart from unwanted pregnancies, many adolescents are also putting themselves at risk of contracting sexually transmitted diseases, including HIV infection. Health promotion in the field of sexual health should however take into account the potential pressures upon adolescents from peers and society in general which, over the last 30 years, has taken a liberal view towards sexual permissiveness. Adolescents may feel they are being coerced into becoming sexually active in order to confirm their masculinity or femininity (Parry-Jones 1985). Mcfarlane and Mcpherson (1992) suggest that health promoters should be aware of the wide range of adolescent attitudes towards sexual activity. Apart from pressures on adolescents to become sexually active there may be cognitive and cultural problems in trying to promote sexual health. We have already referred to the difficulties that adolescents may have in understanding abstract concepts and comprehending the consequences of sexual activity may be beyond the cognitive abilities of some adolescents. In addition, there may be cultural objections to the discussion of sexuality, particularly in mixed gender groups. The 1986 Education Act put the responsibility of deciding whether sexual health should be taught on individual schools, and on the parents whose children make up the school population (Scowen 1988), although a DFE directive (Cohen 1994) now makes it mandatory. What this amounted to was that some adolescents were not taught about sexual health at all, and others may be limited in the information they were allowed to receive. Clearly, the area of promoting sexual health is complex, but serves as one example of how primary preventive health care can be problematic and ultimately unsuccessful.

Secondary prevention

Health promotion is also concerned with secondary prevention, which is aimed at individuals with asymptomatic disease. Examples of secondary preventive activity during adolescence are screening for vision and hearing defects, regular dental inspection, the early detection of eating disorders, depression and sexually transmitted disease and other activities which involve detecting asymptomatic disease. Clearly school nurses are at the forefront of secondary prevention in relation to school-aged adolescents, but practice nurses and hospital-based nurses are also frequently involved in screening and detection. The aim of health promoters must be to encourage adolescents to take responsibility for their own health (Ewles and Simnett 1992), which should include giving information about how to gain access to screening and the purpose of screening. Health promotion should emphasize the positive benefits of taking such responsibility rather than focusing on the negative. For example, in relation to dental health, whilst adolescents should be given information about the effects of tooth decay, emphasis should be placed upon how good you feel about yourself after you've been for a check-up or finished your dental treatment. Encouraging the internal administration of reinforcement for health seeking behaviour is a useful strategy for strengthening positive actions.

We must ensure however that secondary preventive services are accessible to adolescents if we are to encourage them to utilize such services. For example, if an adolescent is worried about the possibility of having contracted a sexually transmitted disease, it may be difficult for that adolescent to seek help if clinics only operate in the evenings on weekdays. We have already referred to the benefits of school nurses running 'surgeries' in school where students can seek information from the nurse in confidence about a range of issues. Such surgeries should have available information about where and when various clinics operate. A further useful strategy which some further and higher education establishments have adopted is the siting of regular sexual health clinics on campus, which can offer practical assistance and advice about contraception, sexually transmitted diseases and pregnancy etc.

Tertiary prevention

Tertiary prevention involves the maintenance or improvement of health in people who are not healthy, by the prevention of avoidable complications of chronic illness or disability. For some adolescents, existing childhood problems continue into adolescence, whilst for others adolescence marks the beginning of a chronic health problem. Health professionals working with adolescents will inevitably encounter a wide range of need in relation to chronic ill health. These needs are often complicated by the physiological and psychological changes which occur during this period, as well as the move towards independence. The enhanced cognitive abilities of the adolescent with cystic fibrosis, for example, give greater personal insight into health status but also require that the adolescent faces up to the realities of the future and their own mortality (Taylor 1994). Some adolescents find that their health deteriorates markedly during this period and they find it difficult to keep up with their healthy peers. For example, staying the weekend with friends or going on extended school trips can be complicated if not impossible.

Tertiary prevention with adolescents who have chronic health problems is complex, and must take into account the nature of ill health or disability in the context of psychological and physiological development. Because of the very specific nature of problems, tertiary prevention is best carried out on a one-to-one basis, whether the adolescent is at school, in hospital or at home. Information about how to prevent the complications of ill health should of course account for the cognitive abilities of the adolescent. We have already stressed the importance of getting to know adolescents before trying to impart information and this point applies equally in terms of tertiary prevention. Taylor (1994) suggests that it is important to assess previous knowledge and understanding, but that it is also necessary to address obvious anger or aggressive feelings the adolescent may have because it will otherwise be a barrier to communication. Information given to the adolescent should be appropriate in terms of the adolescent's language, age and culture, and should be backed up with written information if possible.

Finally, in relation to adolescents with chronic ill health or disability, it is always important to remember that adolescents like to 'belong' and be able to identify with a peer group. The adolescent who has to wear a brace for scoliosis, the diabetic who needs to inject insulin regularly, the epileptic who cannot get a provisional driving licence, and many adolescents with specific problems can find themselves isolated from their peers because of the restrictions of their health. This potential isolation can contribute to non-compliance with treatment regimens and further complications. Perhaps one of the most important aims of tertiary prevention with adolescents is to explore their coping strategies and to help adolescents to develop further adaptive ways of coping. Eiser (1990), in an excellent review of research into the needs of children and adolescents with chronic disease, suggests that adaptation can be improved by increasing disease-related knowledge and by developing the social skills of the adolescent. For example, the diabetic adolescent may be very capable of managing treatment at home, but may benefit from exploration of how to cope with treatment in different situations. Working through imagined and real fears in relation to coping in different situations can enhance social skills and lead to greater confidence in personal abilities to cope.

The implications for nurses

We have referred, throughout this chapter, to examples of how nurses can positively influence the health behaviour of adolescents. Whilst particular nurses clearly have a role to play in health promotion, it should be seen as part of the role of every nurse regardless of the client group they work with or the setting in which they carry out their work. It is encouraging that health promotion is currently being given a higher profile in nurse education programmes and that nurses are seeing it more and more as an integral part of their role. However, if nurses are to be effective promoters of health, particularly with children and adolescents, it is important for them to understand the psychosocial influences which impinge on the worlds of their clients, and to recognize the importance of learning and cognitive development when they are planning health promotion strategies.

References

Bandura, A. (1977) *Social Learning Theory*. Prentice-Hall, New Jersey.

Beard, R.M. (1969) *An Outline of Piaget's Developmental Psychology*. Routledge and Kegan Paul, London.

Botvin, G. (1984) The Life Skills Training Model: a broad spectrum approach to the prevention of cigarette smoking. In: *Health Education and Youth*. (Ed. G. Campbell). Falmer Press, London.

Bowie, C. and Ford, N. (1989) Sexual behaviour of young people and the risk of HIV infection. *Journal of Epidemiology and Community Health*, 43(1): 61–65.

Burkist, W. and Gerbing, D.W. (1990) *Psychology: Boundaries and Frontiers*. Scott, Foresman/Little, Brown, Glenview, Illinois.

Child, D. (1986) *Psychology and the Teacher*, 4th edn. Cassell Education, London.

Cohen, P. (1994) The role of the school nurse in providing sex education. *Nursing Times*, 90(23): 36–38.

Conger, J.J. (1991) *Adolescence and Youth*, 4th edn. Harper Collins, New York.

Curtis, H., Lawrence, C. and Tripp, J. (1989) Teenage sexuality: implications for controlling AIDS. *Archives of Disease in Childhood*, 64: 1240–1245.

Eiser, C. (1990) Psychological effects of chronic disease. *Journal of Child Psychology and Psychiatry*, 31(1): 85–98.

Elkind, D. and Bowen, R. (1979) Imaginary audience behaviour in children and adolescents. *Developmental Psychology*, 15: 38–44.

Ewles, I. and Simnett, L. (1992) *Promoting Health: A Practical Guide*, 2nd edn. Scutari Press, London.

French, J. (1984) Health education and youth: whose responsibility? In: *Health Education and Youth*. (Ed. G. Campbell). Falmer Press, London.

Gibson, M. (1987) Developing what used to be 'the soft option'. *Health at School*, 2(4): 116–117.

Hersov, L. (1985) Adoption and fostering. In: *Child and Adolescent Psychiatry*, 2nd edn. (Eds M. Rutter and L. Hersov). Blackwell Scientific Publications, Oxford.

Keating, D.P. (1980) Thinking processes in adolescence. In: *Handbook of Adolescent Psychiatry*. (Ed. J. Adelson). John Wiley, New York.

Kolbe, L.J. (1984) Improving the health of children and youth: frameworks for behavioural research and development. In: *Health Education and Youth*. (Ed. G. Campbell). Falmer Press, London.

Lovell, K. (1961) A follow-up study of Inhelder and Piaget's 'The growth of logical thinking'. *British Journal of Psychology*, 52: 143–154.

Macfarlane, A. and Mcpherson, A. (1992) Sex and teenagers. *Health Visitor*, 65(1): 18–19.

Moriasy, J. and Thomas, L. (1990) *Triple Jeopardy – Women and AIDS*. Panos Books.

Muller, D.J., Harris, P.J., Wattley, L. and Taylor, J. (1992) *Nursing Children: Psychology, Research and Practice*, 2nd edn. Chapman and Hall, London.

Overton, W.F., Ward, S.L., Noveck, I.A., Black, J. and O'Brien, D.P. (1987) Form and content in the development of deductive reasoning. *Developmental Psychology*, 23: 22–30.

Parry-Jones, W.L. (1985) Adolescent disturbance. In: *Child and Adolescent Psychiatry*, 2nd edn. (Ed. M. Rutter and L. Hersov). Blackwell Scientific Publications, Oxford.

Reid, D. (1984) The contribution of school health education programmes to health and education. In: *Health Education and Youth*. (Ed. G. Campbell). Falmer Press, London.

Schools Council/Health Education Council (1982) *Health Education 13–18*. Forbes Publications, London.

Scowen, P. (1988) AIDS education in schools: how to put the message across. *Health at School*, 3(5) 142–145.

Stewart, A.J. and Orme, J. (1991) Why do adolescents smoke? In *Child Care: Some Nursing Perspectives*. (Ed. A. Glasper). Wolfe, London.

Tauer, K.M. (1983) Promoting effective decision making in sexually active adolescents. *Nursing Clinics of North America*, 18(2): 275–292.

Taylor, J. (1994) The sick and well adolescent. In: *Health Promotion and Patient Education*. (Ed. P. Webb). Chapman and Hall, London.

Tones, K., Tilford, S. and Robinson, Y. (1990) *Health Education Effectiveness and Efficiency*. Chapman and Hall, London.

Further reading

Burnard, P. (1992) *Counselling: a Guide to Practice in Nursing*. Butterworth Heinemann, Oxford.

This useful book provides guidance for working in group situations.

Campbell, G. (ed) (1984) *Health Education and Youth*. Falmer Press, London.

This comprehensive book covers a wide range of health education perspectives with useful examples which are relevant to health professionals working with adolescents.

Child, D. (1986) *Psychology and the Teacher*, 4th edn. Cassell Education, London.

Although this book is written for teachers, the chapters on learning theory and practice (Chapter 5), and on concept formation and cognitive development (Chapter 7) are very useful in that they discuss the application of psychological theory to practice.

Gross, R.D. (1992) *Psychology: The Science of Mind and Behaviour*, 2nd edn. Hodder and Stoughton, London.

Chapter 7 of this excellent book provides a useful synopsis on learning theory.

Chapter 6
Adolescent Health Care

Adolescence is a time of life that is usually associated with good physical and mental health. However, good health is not universal during this period, and many adolescents will come into contact with the health services because of acute or chronic health problems, which either commence during adolescence or which have arisen during childhood and continue to be problematic during adolescence.

One of the great debates of contemporary paediatrics relates to adolescents and hospital services. Adolescence is rarely viewed as a specialty in its own right, particularly when health problems are physical in nature. The debate revolves around where adolescents should be nursed when they are admitted to hospital, and whether they should be cared for by paediatricians or specialist adult-oriented doctors. Most of us agree that ideally adolescents should be cared for in adolescent units with specially trained staff who are fully conversant with their particular needs. However, the health services do not exist within an ideal world, and are constantly trying to balance the limited available resources for the provision of health care. Specialist units for adolescents are rare and the debate continues.

Regardless of where adolescents are nursed in hospital, or whether care is delivered in hospital or the community, adolescents who have health problems can find that life is particularly traumatic. The normal tasks of adolescence (see Chapter 4), which can pose enormous difficulties for well adolescents, can be complicated by physical or mental ill health, whether illness is acute or chronic in nature. Even adolescents who have a longstanding health problem which has continued from childhood, may find that medical regimens which have been a familiar and routine part of their lives, are suddenly restrictive and inconvenient as they strive for independence and autonomy.

This chapter will therefore take as its focus three interrelating themes. The first theme will look at adolescent health status, and certain specific areas of concern will be more fully explored in the following four chapters. The second theme relates to where adolescents should be cared for and explores two debates, the first of which is the adult/

children's ward dilemma, and the second the hospital/community dilemma. The final theme relates to the specific needs of adolescents who have acute or recurring physical and mental health problems, and will discuss how best nurses can meet those needs.

Health problems during adolescence

We have already mentioned in the introduction to this chapter that adolescence is a period of life which is commonly associated with good health rather than with health problems. This may account for the lack of attention paid to adolescent ill health by health professionals, although certain health problems have been well researched, such as eating disorders (see Chapter 7). The lack of data may also reflect the lack of common practice about who should care for adolescents with health problems. In terms of nursing research, adolescents are frequently admitted to adult wards but do not comprise a significant number of admissions in relation to other groups. As a group they tend to be excluded from nursing research, possibly because of the small numbers involved, but also because their stage of psychological development may be seen as an uncontrollable extraneous variable. On paediatric wards, similar methodological difficulties may exclude them from inclusion in research activities.

Adolescent morbidity

In total, adolescents use health services far less than younger children and reasons for use also change. In terms of physical disorder, trauma is a major cause of mortality during adolescence and accidental injuries account for a significant number of adolescent admissions (DoH 1992). So too, do disorders of the digestive system such as appendicitis. Malignant conditions such as leukaemia, lymphomas, central nervous system tumours, and bone tumours, whilst rare may also arise during adolescence and account for a large proportion of admissions (Thompson 1990). Health problems emanating from childhood may also necessitate hospital admission, or involvement with acute health care services within the community. Cystic fibrosis, diabetes and juvenile rheumatoid arthritis are examples of such problems.

In terms of psychological disorders during adolescence, Steinberg (1987) suggests that 'misbehaviour' accounts for approximately 20% of referrals, 'serious misbehaviour' (including violence, fire-setting, and drug abuse) and school non-attendance both account for 10% of referrals, threatened or attempted self-injury account for 10–15% of referrals, concern about mood (including anxiety, misery, withdrawal and eating problems) account for 40% of referrals and further opinion requests account for 10–20% of referrals. The most frequent clinical diagnosis is mood disorder, followed by conduct disorder, problems of personality development, schizophrenia and affective psychoses, anorexia and bulimia nervosa, enuresis, encopresis, tics, hysterical disorder, autism and brain disorders (including epilepsy).

As with all 'paediatric' admissions, most health problems requiring hospital admission during adolescence are non-routine emergency admissions (Audit Commission 1993). This may further complicate the debate about where adolescents should be nursed, as time cannot be taken during the pre-admission phase to consider whether, in the absence of specialist facilities, an individual adolescent should best be nursed with adults or with children. This debate is further considered during the next section.

Caring for adolescents in hospital and the community

During the introduction to this chapter we alluded to the debate about where adolescents should be nursed when they require admission to hospital. The debate has been live for some 30 years with the *Platt Report* (1959) first making reference to the need for specialist facilities for adolescent patients. The *Court Report* (1976) also concluded that:

> 'adolescents have needs and problems sufficiently distinguishable from those on the one hand of children and on the other of adults to warrant consideration as a distinct group for health care provision'. (p163)

Such specialist facilities are however almost as rare today as they were then. The Audit Commission (1993) reported that only one in ten of the localities visited during their survey, which investigated children's health services, had separate wards for adolescents, although some had separate areas within the children's wards for adolescent patients. In the absence of such facilities adolescents are either admitted to children's wards or more usually to adult wards. Thornes (1987) reported that 62% of 12–16 year olds receive care on wards which were designated as adult facilities. On adult wards, and on children's wards to a lesser extent, adolescents are likely to be cared for by nurses who have very little formal training in the special needs of this group (Blunden 1989; Gillies 1992). The suitability of such environments is questionable as we will discuss in the following section.

Hospital admission for physical health problems

It is perhaps worthy that, whilst adolescent health care is under-researched, a great deal of attention has at least been placed upon the environment best suited to adolescents who require hospital admission. Burr (1993), in a small study of adolescents and the ward environment, interviewed adolescents who were receiving care on either adult or children's wards. Comments from adolescents being cared for on adult designated wards showed them to be dissatisfied with the elderly population in the ward, the lack of cleanliness and maintenance, and being in a mixed gender ward. They also reported feeling lonely, bored and frightened of both other patients (comments were made about old people moaning and dying), and of their own treatment. They also missed the companionship of adolescents of their own age.

Burr (1993) found that the adolescents being cared for on children's wards were also less than satisfied with the environment, and commented on the lack of privacy, the need to talk with people of their own age, the length of the beds (which were too short), and bed time at 7.30 in the evening. These adolescents also reported feeling isolated at times, and felt that the ward was oriented to younger children. Burr concluded from these data that the children's ward was a more suitable environment, although we must caution that this study involved only a small number of adolescents from one location, and results should not be generalized. Neither did the findings of the study fully support Burr's conclusions as both groups of adolescents expressed dissatisfaction.

Burr's findings, if not her conclusions, are supported by other data however. Shelley (1993) suggests that adult wards give adolescents frightening impressions of illness, whereas children's wards were noisy and provided insufficient privacy. Gillies (1992) also postulated that adolescents find children's wards unsuitable, particularly if they cannot be placed in single rooms. She suggests that being in a bed (again often too short) next to young children and babies leads to some distress. This distress is vividly described by Daniel Steven (1992), a 14-year-old who was admitted to a children's ward for surgery. He described his return from the operating department to the ward:

'Back on Franklin Ward, all is noise. The TV is on, the room is full of Lego, tired looking mothers and two-year-olds who pee on the floor.' (p30)

Sadly, distress appears to be the lasting memory that some adolescents have of hospital admission. Denholm (1990) found in a study of adolescents' memories of hospital four years after discharge that recollec-

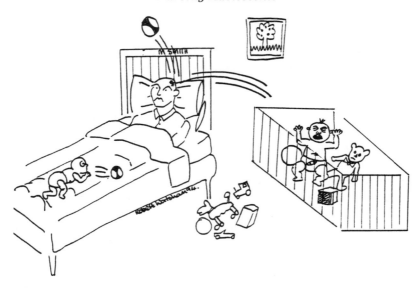

Fig. 6.1   For an adolescent, being in a bed next to children and babies can lead to some distress.

tions of admission tended to focus upon the environment and the loneliness, boredom, depression and fear. They also remembered the lack of privacy and their need to have time on their own, as well as the inevitable two-year-olds!

The conclusion from these studies appears to be that neither adult nor children's wards are ideally suited to the needs of adolescents who require hospitalization. In the absence of a designated adolescent unit the compromise must surely be to assess individual adolescents and make an informed judgement about whether they should be admitted to an adult or a children's ward. This assessment should include detail about the age range of children currently resident on the children's ward, and the wishes of the adolescent. This type of assessment may also be relevant even when adolescent facilities are available. Blunden (1989), in her study which looked at where adolescents would *prefer* to be nursed, found that 80.8% of 11-year-olds preferred to be nursed on the children's ward, rather than on an adolescent unit, whereas 100% of 13-year-olds preferred the adolescent unit. Age may not, however, be a totally reliable determinant of choice. Previous experiences of hospitalization, particularly when adolescents have a long history of repeated admissions, may result in them being unwilling to give up the secure and familiar environment of the children's ward. In these situations adolescents have frequently developed trusting relationships with nursing and other staff, and are unwilling to exchange this familiarity for something which may, or may not be better. Individual assessment must then form the basis for deciding where care will be delivered, and the success of that assessment should be carefully evaluated throughout the adolescent's time in hospital. It may be that initial decisions based on data available at the time of admission need to be reviewed, and the adolescent moved to a more suitable environment. Finally, to conclude this section it is worth reiterating the views of Thompson (1990) which have relevance to nurses caring for adolescents, whether on a children's ward, an adult ward or an adolescent unit:

> 'Adolescent patients must be cared for not as children or adults but as an age group with specific needs. It is important to understand their development and how medical problems affect their mood, behaviour and coping. It is a special time in their lives, both psychologically and biologically. They need and deserve a special kind of understanding.' (p138)

Hospital admission for mental health problems

We have, for purposes of clarity, separated physical reasons for hospital admissions from admission for psychiatric disorder. Whilst it is a convenient division, particularly as hospital services remain to a great extent divided in terms of the types of disorder they provide for, it is important to recognize that physical and psychological disorder frequently co-exist. Graham and Rutter (1973) found in their Isle of Wight study that children and adolescents with physical disorders were two and a half times more likely to have psychiatric disorders, than were children with no physical disorder. Similarly, in a later study by McGee and Stanton (1990), an association was found between anxiety disorders and respiratory/allergic conditions. Whether physical disorders represent risk factors for the development of psychiatric disorder or vice versa is unclear. What is evident however, is that nurses caring predominantly for children and adolescents with physical disorders, and those caring for children and adolescents with psychiatric disorders, are likely to encounter disorders for which they were not specifically trained.

The development of hospital services for adolescents with psychiatric disorder and physical disorder have followed a similar pattern. The first psychiatric units for adolescents were founded in the late 1940s, with in-patient treatment prior to that time being largely provided by the large general psychiatric institutions, and out-patient care being provided by the child guidance clinics and in clinics within special departments of general psychiatric hospitals (Steinberg 1987). However, in 1976 the Court Report found that in spite of the existence of special units, provision for adolescents remained sparse and that 'too many adolescents are unsuitably placed on adult psychiatric wards' (p270). The later review of services for adolescents with psychiatric disorder *Bridges Over Troubled Waters* (Health Advisory Service 1986) also found discrepancies in provision and gaps in provision which were unacceptable and resulted in adolescents being cared for in unsuitable environments. More recently, the Department of Health (1991), in their report *The Welfare of Children and Young People in Hospital,* have reiterated that children and adolescents who develop serious mental health problems which require in-patient hospital care should be admitted to specialist units where they can receive care from appropriately qualified staff.

The reasons for providing special facilities for adolescents with psychiatric disorder are in many ways similar to the rationale for providing adolescent facilities in general hospitals. There are, however, important therapeutic advantages to segregating adolescents from adult in-patients in psychiatric units. These advantages relate to the inclusion of the family in therapy which can be difficult if the environment is not designed or adapted to promote family therapy. A second reason which cannot be ignored relates to the problems of negative behaviours which can, in effect, be 'learned' from adult role models. Whilst in-patient care was originally thought of as a means of segregating young people from adverse family circumstances (Hersov and Bentovim 1985), and there is little doubt that external factors (including school and the family) contribute to psychiatric problems during adolescence (Steinberg 1987), the fundamental focus of care is to help the adolescent and family to overcome personal and social problems and return to a more normal life within the community. Achieving this goal involves complex multidisciplinary support from health, social and educational agencies.

Community services for adolescents with physical and psychological disorder

Whilst there is clearly a view that adolescents who require in-patient hospital care should be afforded special facilities, there is overriding opinion that hospital admission should be the last resort and where possible care should be provided within the community. For nearly 40 years psychologists have warned of the detrimental effects of hospitalization on children (Bowlby 1951; Robertson and Robertson 1971; Wolff 1973; Douglas 1975). In addition, both the *Platt Report* (1959) and the *Court Report* (1976) advocated the provision of community nursing services as an alternative to hospital admission for some children because of the potential adverse psychological effect of admission. It was, however, not until the early 1990s that paediatric community nursing care provision became a reality in a major way, although provision still remains sporadic. The Royal College of Nursing have produced a register of provision which shows that some areas remain without any comprehensive provision (see RCN 1993).

Accounts of the work of paediatric community nursing teams (Atwell and Gow 1985; Dryden 1986, 1989a, 1989b; Campbell 1987; Kitson *et al.* 1987; Glasper *et al.* 1989; Sidey 1990) also show great variation in the work undertaken by nurses, both in terms of diagnostic criteria and the ages of patients. We can find no evidence of paediatric community nursing teams who provide specifically focused services for adolescents in the community. It is unclear as to whether this is because the need does not exist for such services, which seems doubtful, or whether services do exist but those involved in such services have not communicated their work.

Community nursing services for adolescents with psychiatric disorder also appear to be limited and sporadic (Health Advisory Service 1986), although there are specialist services in existence (Hinks *et al.* 1988; McMorrow 1990). Community psychiatric nursing services have a longer and more structured history than do paediatric community nursing services, and there is also a recognized English National Board course and career structure for community psychiatric nurses. However, it is unlikely that either mental health or children's nurses will have had sufficient education in adolescent care, unless they have undertaken further study after qualification. Our own informal investigation as to whether changes in nurse education over the last five years will have increased the emphasis placed upon adolescents show that it is unlikely. There is clearly a need for more education either in pre-registration training or after registration for those nurses who are working with adolescents in the community as well as in hospital. As Blunden (1989) suggests, 'nurse training needs to be adjusted to cope with adolescents *en masse*' (p13).

It has not been our intention here to criticize those services which are providing care for adolescents in the community, but rather to suggest that if adolescents are to be considered as a special and distinctive group of clients then there must be coverage, in terms of the provision of services, as well as education for those nurses involved·in adolescent care. We suggest that Regional Health Authorities must place greater emphasis on funding additional training, and be prepared to fund research into the specific focus of community services.

The provision of services

The final theme which we will discuss in this chapter relates to the provision of services and how nurses can provide care which meets defined need. We have already discussed where adolescents should be nursed and have suggested the need to ensure that adolescents are not admitted to hospital unless there is no alternative. There will however, always be a need to admit some adolescents to hospital and it is to the nature of hospital provision that we now turn. The National Association for the Welfare of Children in Hospital (now renamed Action for Sick Children) published a set of standards for the provision of care to adolescents in hospital upon which we have based our discussion. The Action for Sick Children statement on adolescents in hospital is given in Table 6.1.

Table 6.1   Action for Sick Children Policy Paper 3: Adolescents in Hospital

Action for Sick Children believes that

Adolescent patients have their own special needs

Staff caring for adolescents should be aware of the emotional, intellectual and social as well as physical needs of this age group

Adolescents should be nursed in a self-contained area which forms part of the paediatric unit

Adolescents should be provided with facilities to continue with their education, as far as they are able, whilst they are in hospital

How to achieve this

Planning, building and adapting hospitals

Facilities for adolescents should be planned (service and capital as a complete unit, including in-patient and day care, but excluding out-patient provision)

Adolescent out-patients should be seen in the clinic appropriate to their problem

Upgrading and adaption of existing services and accommodation should take into account the special needs of adolescents

Staff caring for adolescents

Staff, including those in out-patient departments, should be trained in the psychological care of adolescents, especially their needs of privacy, confidentiality, independence, self-responsibility and information concerning their wellbeing and treatment

There should be available to each adolescent ward the services of a psychologist or group leader trained in group work with adolescents. Regular group meetings should be organized

Education staff should provide programmes suited to the needs of each individual adolescent, to minimize disruption of educational progress

Reproduced by kind permission of Action for Sick Children

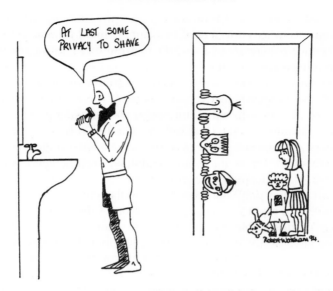

Fig. 6.2 Adolescents may need more privacy than they can find in a children's ward.

Adolescents have a greater need for privacy than younger children (MacKenzie 1988; Audit Commission 1993) and require, particularly, separate washing and toilet areas which afford privacy (DoH 1991; Kelly 1991; Gillies 1992). Nurses should be aware that adolescents may feel embarrassed about their bodies and should anticipate their need for privacy. While it is sensible practice to supervise younger children in the bath, for example, it is clearly unacceptable practice with adolescents, unless there is a special reason to do so.

Peer company is also very important to adolescents and contact with friends outside hospital can be helpful in enabling friends to have some idea of what the ill adolescent is experiencing as well as ensuring that the adolescent in hospital can keep up with what is going on in the outside world. Visits from friends should be encouraged (Shelley 1993), but not forced as not all young people will wish their friends to see them (Kuykendall 1989; Gillies 1992). If friends do visit there should be somewhere that they can meet, preferably with TV, video and music. It is also helpful if the adolescent in hospital has access to kitchen facilities, not only for offering friends a drink, but also so that they can have some control over the structuring of their own time (DoH 1991). It may be necessary to limit such contacts with friends depending upon the adolescent's health status and the status of other occupants on the ward. Setting rules for behaviour and boundaries for the numbers of visitors and the time they can realistically spend visiting is important, and should be negotiated with the adolescent from the outset. Embarrassing confrontations with adolescents in front of their friends about rules which they were unaware of does little to promote a trusting relationship between nurses and patients.

Admission to hospital can be highly detrimental to adolescents in terms of their education. Adolescents should be encouraged, if they are well enough, to keep up with their study, and study facilities should be available (Thompson 1990; DoH 1991; Gillies 1992). Ensuring continuity in terms of educational input may require considerable collaboration between hospital teachers, school teachers, nurses, parents and the adolescent. Many hospital teachers are trained in infant teaching (Save the Children Fund 1989) and hospital schools, which frequently have to accommodate a rapidly changing population of different ages and abilities, may be unsuitable for an adolescent who is, for example, taking Advanced Level study. It is much more appropriate for teachers from the adolescent's school to keep a watchful eye on the adolescent's study. This has the added advantage of familiarizing the teachers with the adolescent's health problems which can be helpful when the adolescent returns to school.

One of the recurring themes of this book is the growing need for independence and autonomy during adolescence and we have discussed independence in relation to health status in Chapter 2. When adolescents are admitted to hospital, independence and autonomy should be promoted. This means ensuring that adolescent patients are involved in planning, and making decisions about their own care and treatment (Jordan and Kelfer 1983; Kelly 1991; Gillies 1992), although nurses should be aware that legislation in relation to consent during adolescence is extremely complex (see Chapter 1).

The process of involving adolescents in care should begin during the assessment and be reflected in the care plan which should clearly reflect the wishes of the adolescent. It is important for nurses to be aware, in relation to assessment, that adolescents may wish some of their experiences and feelings to remain confidential, even from their parents. Granting, wherever possible, the confidentiality expected by adult patients is an important part of the process of providing effective care. Assessment should, therefore, be carried out both with and without the presence of parents.

Part of the process of promoting independence and autonomy in hospital relates also to the delivery of care particularly in adolescents who have on-going health problems. Whilst it is acknowledged that poor compliance with medical regimens may precipitate admission in some cases (Hentigen and Kungas 1992; Tameroff *et al.* 1992) there is no evidence to suggest that forcing adolescents to become dependent on nurses or parents has any effect on future compliance. It also seems detrimental to the promotion of self-care in adolescents who are complying with treatments, to make them dependent on nursing staff for the administration of medication which they normally control when they are at home. We can find little evidence relating to self-administration of medication in hospital by adolescents (although we are aware of trials in progress), and suggest that with careful thought in relation to the safety of other patients, self-medication is realistic for some adolescents in hospital. Litman and Shapiro (1992), in one study of self-administration of oral opoids for chronic pain, found that with careful selection of adolescents they could successfully manage their analgesia regimens in hospitals.

As a caveat to the promotion of independence in adolescents with chronic health problems we should perhaps remember that not all adolescents will be prepared or able to accept independence, just as some parents may not feel able to give up the control they have over medical regimens. It is never easy when a child has a chronic health problem, and where medical regimens have provided a structure around which all other family activities have revolved. Whilst some parents may welcome the fact that their child is at last taking some responsibility for their health, others may feel a sense of loss, as well as being fearful that the adolescent won't be able to cope. During periods of hospitalization nurses can find themselves in a difficult position, and should encourage all parties to talk about their feelings. It may be that it is *not* an appropriate time to change the dependence/independence balance between parents and an adolescent, but it may be an appropriate time to discuss how and when changes can take place. Alternatively, it may be the case that parents feel that hospital is the appropriate place for adolescents to become more self-caring given that help is at hand if things go wrong. Clearly the only way to find out is to encourage open and honest communication.

The final area we wish to discuss in relation to the provision of services also relates to parents in terms of enabling them to spend time with adolescents in hospital. Whilst adolescents may wish for increasing detachment from parents when they are well, they frequently have an increased need to have their parents with them whilst they are sick (Pazola and Kushner Gerberg 1985). Hospitals should provide accommodation for the parents of adolescents, just as most hospitals provide such facilities for younger children (DoH 1991; Shelley 1993). The report *Parents Staying Overnight in Hospital with their Children* discussed by Sadler (1988) stresses that parents should be informed of the importance of being with their children, particularly at night and that accommodation should be provided for parents of adolescents as well as younger children.

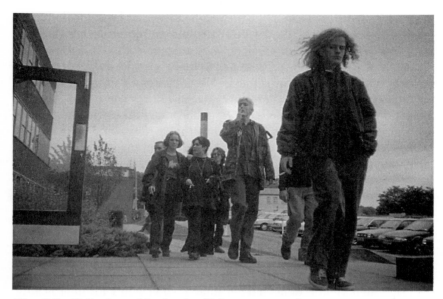

Fig. 6.3 Visits from friends should be encouraged: peer company is very important to adolescents.

The implications for nurses

Caring for adolescents who have physical or mental health problems, whether they are acute or chronic, requires a great deal of skill and understanding. As many parents of adolescents will verify, it is often difficult to predict adolescent behaviour. They tend to be emotionally labile and illness can intensify this lability (Kuykendall 1989). A nurse may feel a trusting relationship has developed with a particular adolescent one day, only to find that the relationship is in shreds the next day, and for no apparent reason.

Whilst we do not wish to be in any way prescriptive we feel it is important to tease out of the knowledge and research reviewed in this chapter a set of guiding principles for caring for adolescents in hospital which relate more to interaction with adolescents than to the structure of services. These principles cannot in any way cover all aspects of caring for adolescents but we hope they may provide a foundation for discussion among nurses who work with adolescents, either constantly or on an intermittent basis:

- independence should be promoted by establishing a trusting relationship and allowing negotiation in care planning;

- ground rules for behaviour should be negotiated and agreed between the adolescent, nurses, parents and other patients;
- nurses must be aware that adolescents may be emotionally labile; learning about the adolescent and being sensitive to mood can guide interaction;
- adolescents need to be able to explore choices as part of their decision making. When reached, decisions should normally be accepted in a value-free way;
- ensure that conversations with adolescents, particularly if they involve giving information, are age, language and culture appropriate;
- address obvious anger and aggression directly – it will be a barrier to communication otherwise.

References

Atwell, J. and Gow, M. (1985) Paediatric trained district nurses in the community: expensive luxury or economic necessity? *British Medical Journal*, 291: 227–229.

Audit Commission (1993) *Children First: A Study of Hospital Services*. HMSO, London.

Blunden, R. (1989) An artificial state. *Paediatric Nursing*, 1(1): 12–13.

Bowlby, J. (1951) *Maternal Care and Mental Health*. WHO, Geneva.

Burr, S. (1993) Adolescents and the ward environment. *Paediatric Nursing*, 5(1): 10–13.

Campbell, M. (1987) Children with ongoing health needs. *Nursing Series*, 23: 871–875.

Court, S.D.M. (1976) *Fit for the Future: Report of the Committee on Child Health Services. Vols I and II*. HMSO, London.

Denholm, C. (1990) Memories of adolescent hospitalization: results from a 4 year follow up study. *CHC*, 19(2): 101–105.

Department of Health (1991) *Welfare of Children and Young People in Hospital*. HMSO, London.

Department of Health (1992) *The Health of the Nation*. HMSO, London.

Department of Health (1993) *The Health of the Nation. Key Area Handbook. Accidents*. HMSO, London.

Douglas, J.W.B. (1975) Early hospital admissions and later disturbances of behaviour and learning. *Developmental Medicine and Child Neurology*, 17: 456–480.

Dryden, S. (1986) Home healing. *Community Outlook*, October: 25–26.

Dryden, S. (1989a) Care in the Community. *Paediatric Nursing*, October: Vol. I, 19–20.

Dryden, S. (1989b) Paediatric medicine in the community. *Paediatric Nursing*, November: Vol. I, 17–18.

Gillies, M. (1992) Teenage trauma. *Nursing Times*, 88 (27): 26–29.

Glasper, A., Gow, M. and Yerrell, P. (1989) A family friend. *Nursing Times*, 85(4): 63–75.

Graham, P. and Rutter, M. (1973) Psychiatric disorder in the young adolescent: a follow up study. *Proceedings of the Royal Society of Medicine*, 66: 1226–1229.

Health Advisory Service (1986) *Bridges Over Troubled Waters*. HMSO, London.

Hentingen, M. and Kungas, H. (1992) Compliance of young diabetics with health regimens. *Journal of Advanced Nursing*, 17: 530–536.

Hersov, L. and Bentovim, A. (1985) In-patient and day-hospital units. In: *Child and Adolescent Psychiatry: Modern Approaches*, 2nd edn. (Eds M. Rutter and L. Hersov). Blackwell Scientific Publications, Oxford.

Hinks, M., Crosbie, C., Adams, M., Skinner, A., Cooper, G. and King, M. (1988) Not child's play. *Nursing Times*, 84(38): 42–44.

Jordan, D. and Kelfer, L.S. (1983) Adolescent potential for participation in health care. *Issues in Comprehensive Paediatric Nursing*, 6:147–156.

Kelly, J. (1991) Caring for adolescents. *Professional Nurse*, June: 498–501.

Kitson, A., Atkinson, B. and Ferguson, B. (1987) Specialist delivery of care. *Nursing Times*, 83(19): 36–40.

Kuykendall, J. (1989) Teenage trauma. *Nursing Times*, 85(27): 26–28.

Litman, R.S. and Shapiro, B.S. (1992) Oral patient-controlled analgesia in adolescents. *Journal of Pain and Symptom Management*, 7(2): 78–81.

MacKenzie, H. (1988) Teenagers in hospital. *Nursing Times*, 84(32): 58–61.

McGee, R. and Stanton, N. (1990) Parent reports of disability among 13 year olds with DSM-III disorders. *Journal of Child Psychology and Psychiatry*, 31(5): 793–801.

McMorrow, R. (1990) The new clinicians. *Senior Nurse*, 10(3): 22–27.

National Association for the Welfare of Children in Hospital (1990) *Setting Standards for Adolescents in Hospital*. NAWCH, London.

Pazola, K. and Kushner Gerberg, A. (1985) Teen Group: a forum for the hospitalized adolescent. *American Journal of Maternal Child Health Nursing*, 10: 265–269.

Platt, H. (1959) *The Welfare of Children in Hospital: Report of the Committee on Child Health Services*. HMSO, London.

Robertson, J. and Robertson, J. (1971) Young children in brief separations: a fresh look. *Psychoanalytic Study of the Child*, 26: 262–315.

Royal College of Nursing (1993) *Directory of Paediatric Community Nursing Services*, 10th edn. RCN, London.

Sadler, S. (1988) Being there. *Nursing Times*, 84(34): 19.

Save the Children Fund (1989) Play provision in hospital. *Paediatric Nursing*, 1(3): 19–20.

Shelley, H. (1993) Adolescent needs in hospital. *Paediatric Nursing*, 5(9): 16–18.

Sidey, A. (1990) Co-operation in care. *Paediatric Nursing*, 2(3): 10–12.

Steinberg, D. (1987) *Basic Adolescent Psychiatry*. Blackwell Scientific Publications, Oxford.

Steven, D. (1992) Like it or lump it. *Nursing Times*, 88(27): 30.

Tameroff, M.H., Festa, R.S., Adesman, A.R. and Walco, G.A. (1992) Therapeutic adherence to oral medication regimens by adolescents with cancer: clinical and psychologic correlates. *Journal of Paediatrics*, 120(5): 812–816.

Thompson, J. (1990) The adolescent with cancer. In: *The Child with Cancer – Nursing Care.* (Ed. J. Thompson). Scutari Press, London.

Thornes, R. (1987) *Where are the Children ?* Caring for Children in the Health Services, London.

Wolff, S. (1973) *Children Under Stress.* Penguin, Harmondsworth.

Further reading

Department of Health (1993) *The Health of the Nation. Key Area Handbook. Accidents.* HMSO, London.

This one of a series of handbooks sets out clear preventive strategies for reducing accidents among children and adolescents, as well as providing useful statistical data about accidents rates and trends.

Thompson, J. (1990) The adolescent with cancer. In: *The Child with Cancer – Nursing Care.* (Ed. J. Thompson). Scutari Press, London.

The chapter on adolescents and indeed the entire book gives excellent accounts of caring for children with cancer, including physical, psychological and social caring from a family-centred perspective.

Chapter 7
Eating Disorders

Physical appearance is important within most societies for people of all ages. During adolescence self-awareness of physical appearance becomes increased, prompted by rapid, marked and mostly uncontrollable physiological development. Inevitably as changes in height, musculature and bodily fat distribution occur, appearance alters and weight increases. As physiological changes stabilize, most adolescents control their weight, and to some extent their body shape, by a combination of diet and exercise. For some, however, adolescence marks the commencement of the exacerbation of eating disorders, the effects of which can be serious, permanent and in some cases life-threatening. The role of the nurse in relation to eating disorders during adolescence is discussed in more depth later in this chapter. However, nurses working in a variety of situations will encounter adolescents with eating disorders. It is somewhat disappointing, therefore, to find that the research basis for nursing adolescents with this range of disorders is limited, particularly in view of the expanding research base emerging from other disciplines. It is to be hoped that this state of affairs will change, since eating disorders are significant both in terms of their prevalence and their impact upon the lives of affected adolescents and their families.

Nutrition in adolescence

The increase in physical growth and energy expenditure during adolescence requires a diet which is high in energy and protein-based foods. The daily requirements depend largely upon physical size, rate of growth, activity levels and gender, with adolescent boys usually having greater nutritional needs than girls. The foods that comprise the diet during adolescence, as at other stages of the lifespan, have important effects upon health and there is evidence which suggests that dietary patterns during adolescence persist into adulthood (see Conger 1991) and can influence later health status, particularly in relation to heart disease (Black 1983; McNamara, 1986).

It is not the intention here to provide guidance as to what the adolescent should eat in order to meet the daily recommended dietary intake. Several reports, including the *National Advisory Committee on Nutrition Education Report* (HEC 1983) and the *Committee on Medical Aspects of Food Policy Report* (DHSS 1984) adequately provide such information. What is evident, however, is that many adolescents fail to eat a diet that meets their nutritional requirements. Fisher (1990) in her research with 299 14–16-year-olds in schools in the Thames Valley showed that the dietary instincts of subjects lead them towards unbalanced diets rather than diets which are nutritious and wholesome.

Research evidence showing why adolescent eating habits develop as they do is limited although it is apparent from the few studies that do exist in this field that the diet during adolescence is influenced by multiple factors including family diet, cultural and religious background, the types of meals available away from home (e.g. school meals), knowledge about nutrition, social pressure, peer conformity and developing moral values such as concern about the ethics of rearing animals to eat (Fisher 1990; Conger 1991). We know also from research into some adolescent eating disorders, particularly anorexia nervosa (Lask and Bryant-Waugh 1992) and bulimia nervosa (Brown *et al.* 1989) that

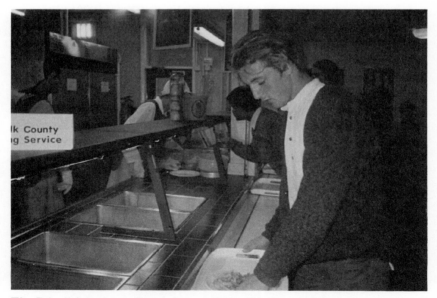

Fig. 7.1 Adolescent eating habits are influenced by multiple factors, including the type of meals available away from home.

anxiety about weight, fear of obesity, distortion of body image, and a strong desire to exert control, can lead the adolescent toward dietary practices which are unsatisfactory. The extent to which these anxieties are present in the non-anorectic and non-bulimic adolescent is as yet unknown but, if such anxieties do exist even to a minor degree, they may well be an additional influence on adolescent dietary habits.

Body image

The fluidity of self-image and anxiety over body image during adolescence has already been discussed in earlier chapters of this book, and the need to conform to the norms of peer groups has been one of the fundamental themes throughout.

The need to conform to the appearance norms of the peer group becomes extremely important during this period, particularly for adolescent girls. The right hairstyle, jewellery, and particularly, the right clothes are all part of belonging to a group, the membership of which becomes increasingly important. The 'right' image for the peer group is frequently one which is derived from advertising in popular magazines and on television, and which reflects stereotypes which look physically attractive and are usually impossibly thin. A study in the United States which looked at obesity in television characters, found that obese characters were never found in commercials and that only 7% of adolescent characters on television were obese (Dietz 1990). Physical attractiveness and thinness are also often portrayed, particularly by the media, as being synonymous with popularity and success. The influence of the media reflects, and contributes to, cultural ideals of thinness which play a major part in the development of adolescents' views of how they should look and how they feel about their own appearance. Fontaine (1991) suggests that the development of eating disorders and subclinical eating disorders can be related to the 'contemporary cultural ideal of thinness' (p669) in many sufferers. Adolescent girls, particularly in early adolescence, are more likely to be dissatisfied with their appearance (Streigel-Moore *et al.* 1986). It has been suggested that this dissatisfaction with appearance, when combined with a cultural ideal of thinness, can contribute to the development of anorexia nervosa or bulimia nervosa, or sub-clinical eating disorder, or result in adolescents being miserable because they are, or perceive themselves to be, overweight (Fontaine 1991).

The relationship between satisfaction with physical appearance and self-esteem is one which probably stems from early childhood. Love and Seaton (1991) suggest that children as young as 7 or 8 learn that obese children are most likely to be teased and left out of games. Children learn to dread being overweight and internalize the culture's hatred and rejection of fatness. Their concept of body size and physical attractiveness comes to match an impossible cultural ideal which, according to Love and Seaton can develop into a weight phobia in adolescence. Swartz (1985) goes even further and defines anorexia nervosa as a culture-bound syndrome which implies that any study of anorexia must consider the social context within which the anorectic is functioning. The concept of normality, in this case relating to ideal weight, is an important consideration and changes from culture to culture. Clearly, however, the cultural ideal of normality and abnormality, influence body image and any subsequent dissatisfaction with that image.

Eating disorders during adolescence

Given the preoccupation with body image and physical attractiveness during adolescence, it is perhaps surprising that more young people do not develop serious eating disorders during this period. However, the influence of peers and the media must be seen within a wider context which includes family influence and greater cognitive abilities. Adolescence does not mean total dependence upon peer groups to the exclusion of previous learning and conflicting influence, nor do all adolescent peer groups crave thinness. However, it is a time when it appears that humans are more susceptible to developing serious eating disorders (Russell 1985).

During adolescence, because of inevitable physical development and growth, weight tends to fluctuate although for most adolescents it will stay within acceptable norms. After growth has stabilized, weight also tends to stabilize. However, in some adolescents problems arise. These problems usually relate to chronic over eating which can lead to, or exacerbate, obesity, to serious under eating, which can result in anorexia nervosa, and to abnormal eating behaviour, bulimia nervosa, which can be preceded by obesity or anorexia nervosa (Russell, 1985).

Obesity

Defining obesity is difficult, and the classification of obesity has tended to vary over time, and within cultures. What is clear is that serious obesity can contribute to medically defined disease in adulthood, such as hypertension and type II diabetes mellitis (Graham 1985). However, when a person is deemed to be obese is less clear (Passmore 1986). The most usual classifications, according to Passmore, are based on the ratio of weight to the square of height, which is refered to as the body mass index (BMI). Various centile charts have been designed for assessing height/weight ratios. Tricep skinfold thickness has also been used as an indicator for obesity and again normative centile charts have been developed (Tanner and Whitehouse 1975).

Obesity in adolescence is more common, by far, than anorexia nervosa or bulimia nervosa (Dietz 1990), and is a problem which often originates in childhood, Stark *et al.* (1981) found, in their longitudinal study, that 40% of overweight 7-year-olds became overweight adults. It is also apparent that obesity during adolescence is increasing. National studies in the United States over a 15 year period from 1965 to 1980 showed an increase in adolescent obesity of 39%, and an increase in superobesity of 64% (see Dietz, 1990). Obesity, was defined in these studies as a tricep skinfold in excess of the 85th percentile, and super-obesity as a tricep skinfold thickness in excess of the 95th percentile. Further analysis of data from these studies showed that increases in obesity were greater among adolescent girls and among white adolescents, although there was a greater increase in prevalence among black adolescents.

The causes of obesity during childhood and adolescence are slowly being investigated and understood but data are confounded by difficulties in classifying when a child or adolescent is 'plump', as opposed to being obese. It does appear however, that 'plumpness' and obesity are both influenced by psychological, biological and social factors.

When exploring psychological influences upon obesity, it is frequently difficult to ascertain whether psychological dysfunction contributes to the development of obesity, or whether it is obesity which results in psychological dysfunctioning. What is apparent is that obese adolescents are often preoccupied with their weight and tend to be socially withdrawn, anxious and sensitive (Kalucy 1976), which Tobias and Gordon (1980) suggest could be associated with the stigma attached to obesity. Whether the obese adolescent reacts to social criticism and stigma is however, according to Conger (1991), dependent upon the state of the adolescent's self-esteem during the transition from childhood to adolescence. Those who have a low self-esteem tend to be more vulnerable to social criticism than those who have gained self-esteem. It is possible, given the number of obese children who continue to be obese during adolescence (Stark *et al.* 1981), that the lack of self-esteem in some adolescents may be associated with criticism and rejection relating to their obesity in childhood. However, there are no available scientifically derived data to support this supposition and clearly there is a need for further research in this important area.

Graham (1985) also suggests that obese adolescents tend to consistently differ from non-obese adolescents in their body image. In common with anorectics, obese adolescents tend to overestimate their body size and shape. This suggestion is interesting in light of studies into body image and obesity. Kaplan and Wadden (1986) found that obesity appears to have no effect on body image in childhood, but an early study of adults who have been obese as adolescents showed strongly distorted body images (Stunkard and Burt 1967).

Social factors which may influence adolescent obesity have also been discussed in the literature but, as with investigations into psychological influences, there is little in the way of sound scientific evidence to support what are mainly anecdotal associations. Early studies (see Graham 1985) suggested that parents may encourage overeating as a way of keeping their children close to them. The prevalence of social and psychological problems in such families was thought to be high. The obese children used eating as a comforting behaviour when faced with stressful situations. Graham goes on to infer that the presence of obesity may represent a mechanism for coping with an otherwise intolerable family situation. Conger (1991) makes similar inferences in relation to the adolescent and other social situations. He suggests that overeating may represent a way of avoiding athletic activities and sexual relationships. Dietz (1990) found that there was a significant relationship between television viewing and obesity in a study of adolescents in the United States; the more television watched by the child and adolescent, the more likely they were to be obese. However, significant correlations can not be used to indicate causal relationships, and it is therefore unclear as to whether watching television leads to obesity or whether obese adolescents, because they are unable or unwilling to take part in other activities, such as sport, resort to filling up their time with watching television.

A further social variable which may influence obesity is socioeconomic status. Obesity is far more common in developed countries in children and adolescents from lower socioeconomic groups (Stunkard 1985). Graham (1985) suggests that this correlation may be associated with breast feeding rates, diet and exercise.

The third possible influence upon obesity in adolescence relates to genetic susceptibility although, as with psychological and sociological influences, evidence is muddled. Certainly the results of early twin studies (see Hawks and Brook 1979) indicated that results could be misleading and uncertainty about genetic influences persisted for the next decade. However, recent studies on identical twins (Bouchard *et al.* 1990; Stunkard *et al.* (1990) have again pointed to an inherited predisposition to obesity. Further evidence which relates to genetic influences in chronic-underweight also adds to the argument that there may be an innate basis for weight (Holland *et al.* 1984).

Obesity is then a significant problem for many adolescents. The causes of obesity remain unclear although psychological, social and biological influences have been implicated. The picture is clouded by the apparent impact of obesity upon psychological and social functioning. Without longitudinal, population-based studies, it is unlikely that a clear view will emerge as to whether psychological and social factors lead to obesity, or whether obesity *per se* leads to psychological and social dysfunctioning. Recent evidence relating to a genetic basis for obesity has added an interesting dimension to the study of obesity, and we can look forward to similar studies being undertaken using larger samples, which can verify these findings. It is possibly that, in the future, susceptible children and adolescents may be identified and interventions designed which can prevent the onset of obesity, and its consequences.

Anorexia nervosa

The second eating disorder which will be discussed in this chapter is anorexia nervosa, which was first described in the late nineteenth century by Gull and Laseque (Showalter 1987). The classical medical definition of 'anorexia' refers to loss of appetite, although it has become apparent that in anorexia nervosa, loss of appetite is not a fundamental feature. The anorectic is often obsessed with food and frequently feels hungry, and it is a fear of weight gain that leads the individual with anorexia nervosa to mimic signs of appetite loss. Anorexia nervosa, then, is more about weight phobia that appetite (Palmer 1980).

Anorexia nervosa, is a condition which is characterized by serious weight loss (Steinberg 1987), caused by food avoidance and sometimes exacerbated by rigorous exercise regimes, purging and vomiting. In addition, the anorectic shows an intense fear of gaining weight, in spite of being severely underweight, demonstrates a distorted body image, and has either primary or secondary amenorrhoea (see Edelstein *et al.* 1989).

Epidemiological data have provided useful information relating to the incidence and prevalence of anorexia nervosa. A comprehensive review of studies investigating anorexia nervosa in the United States showed a range in prevalence among adolescent females ranging from zero to 2.6% (Shisslak *et al.* 1990). Rates for adolescent males ranged from zero to 0.1%. Russell (1985), in a review of incidence and prevalence studies in Britain, cites incidence as ranging between 0.6–1.6 per 100 000 of the whole population, although other studies have found zero prevalence (Johnson-Sabine *et al.* 1988; King 1989). Original reports from the 1970s that anorexia nervosa was a predominantly caucasian disorder have recently been disputed with evidence that children and adolescents from ethnic minorities are also affected (see Lask and Bryant-Waugh 1992). It also appears that prevalence rises among certain groups such as adolescent girls in independent schools, drama students and physical education students (Slade 1984), and ballet students (Garner and Garfinkel 1980). Slade (1984) suggests that there may be an association between the incidence of anorexia nervosa and educational expectations particularly relating to body shape and achievement:

'Where a high value on hard work and professional achievement is explicitly associated with regulation of weight and body shape, this can play a part in the creation of this illness' (p148).

Care must be taken, however, when considering prevalence and incidence in relation to anorexia nervosa. Ledoux *et al.* (1991) suggest that rates may vary because of differences relating to sampling and diagnostic criteria.

As with studies of obesity, psychological, social and biological influences upon anorexia nervosa have been implicated in studies over the last two decades or so, although the psychopathology of anorexia nervosa remains controversial (Gowers *et al.* 1991) due to the complex interaction between psychological and physical factors associated with the disorder (Lask and Bryant-Waugh 1992). Various studies reviewed by Shisslak *et al.* (1990) have reported that anorectic adolescents have lower self-esteem, greater incidences of anxiety, depression, moodiness, and self-doubt, and more negative body images. There is no suggestion that these features are causal in terms of the onset of anorexia nervosa, but rather that they are manifest after onset, although Bruch (1982) suggests that the eating dysfunction results from problems relating to self-concept, identity and autonomy. Whilst anorectics are frequently reported to have been extremely 'good' children they lack a clear sense of identity and emerging selfhood. The family of anorectics are reported to be overcontrolling and constrictive (Shisslak *et al.* 1990) and anorectics have an apparent need to exert control over their own lives. Controlling their own body shape and size, and their diet, are areas where they can successfully exert control (Larson and Johnson 1982). Indeed some anorectics attempt to take over control of the eating habits of the family (Muscari 1988).

An early study by Morgan and Russell (1975) identified predisposing psychological traits in anorectics. Assessment of premorbid personality, based on retrospective information showed that in a sample of 41 anorectics, 68% had abnormal psychological traits including, obsessionality, social anxiety and excessive dependence on the family. In addition, a third of the sample were said to have been overweight as children, and precipitating factors associated with the onset of anorexia nervosa included being teased about being overweight, bereavement and failure at school, although the majority of subjects had an IQ of above the expected mean. Given the association between childhood obesity and low self-esteem reported earlier in this chapter, and the high educational expectations noted in anorectics, the adolescent appears to turn an abundance of anger inwards (Swift *et al.* 1986).

The literature relating to psychological determinants of anorexia nervosa is abundant and often controversial. What is clear, however, is that there is frequently psychological dysfunctioning prior to the onset of anorexia nervosa and that investigation of family background shows a typical pattern of rigidity, lack of communication, denial of conflict and a need for control (Shisslak *et al.* 1990). There is also evidence to suggest that anorexia nervosa is associated with psychological disorder in other family members, and in some anorectics a history of anorexia nervosa in close female relatives (Strober *et al.* 1990). Whether these associations are due to family members living in a similar environment, thus sharing family conflict or whether there is some biological basis for anorexia nervosa is unclear. It is to the innateness theory, that we now turn.

The search for a genetic basis for anorexia nervosa has continued for many years and as with the development of psychological theory, has been subject to controversy. Morgan and Russell (1975) found evidence of psychiatric disorder and anorexia in a small number of their sample, but concluded that these positive family histories probably had more to do with the shared early family environment than heredity. However, Holland *et al.* (1984) in a study of monozygotic and dizygotic twins found that anorexia nervosa occurred more frequently in both monozygotic twins than in dizygotic twins. They concluded that their findings gave at least some weight to the argument that genetic factors play at least some part in the development of anorexia nervosa. Further genetically oriented evidence relates to a genetic impairment of gonadotrophin release from the anterior pituitary gland, and a possible deficit in dopamine feedback (Herzog 1988).

Anorexia nervosa has traditionally been associated with adolescence and young adulthood (see Gowers *et al.* 1991) and Crisp (1980) suggested that its onset may be due to a maladaptive biological response to puberty. However, recent studies have to some extent questioned this theory, as anorexia nervosa has been identified, albeit rarely, in pre-pubertal children (Bryant-Waugh *et al.* 1988; Higgs *et al.* 1989; Gowers *et al* 1991; Lask and Bryant-Waugh 1992). The possibility remains, however, that since changes occur in body fat distribution and hormonal levels for up to three years before the development of secondary sexual characteristics (Taylor 1994) that early onset anorexia nervosa may also be associated with pubertal change. Gowers *et al.* (1991) suggest that in early onset anorexia nervosa the child is anticipating, rather than responding to weight gain typically associated with puberty. In girls with early onset anorexia nervosa, the process of puberty, including menstruation and weight gain is frequently halted which somewhat confounds the influence of puberty upon the development of anorexia nervosa (Lask and Bryant-Waugh 1992).

The association between social determinants and anorexia nervosa is also referred to frequently in the literature, and whilst again there remains contrasting evidence, there is evidence to support this association. High socioeconomic status has long been recognized in relation to anorexia nervosa, with adolescents from social classes I and II being over represented, relative to the population norms (Palmer 1980). Morgan and Russell (1975) found a similar association but remained uncertain as to whether the higher social class was associated with increased causal factors, or whether it reflected differences in help seeking behaviour patterns among this more affluent group. Herzog and Copeland (1985) in a more recent study have however again noted that whilst anorexia nervosa affects all socioeconomic groups, most anorectics are from the middle and upper classes. The reasons for this association are entirely speculative, and revolve around notions of increased pressure to succeed and higher personal expectations. Clearly, further investigation is needed.

A further area of interest in the search for a cause for anorexia nervosa has been family background. Eisele *et al.* (1986) found that anorectics were more likely to come from broken homes and Hsu (1990) suggests that disturbed family relationships are more common in anorectics than in the families of non-anorectics. Russell (1985) suggests that family disruption may precipitate onset. There is, however, no evidence to suggest that family dysfunction is causal, although it does appear to be an important variable.

The role of social influence in the development of eating disorders has already been referred to, and is worthy of mention again in this discussion of anorexia nervosa. We have, for example, already referred to the increased incidence of anorexia nervosa among certain adolescents involved in activities which require them to be slim and fit, such as ballet and drama. In these and other anorectics, identification with a reference group (in this case slim, fit and successful professionals) and the need for a perfect figure becomes strong. Thinness is perceived to be the answer to many of their problems, including early failure in their chosen activity. If the problems do not go away when thinness is achieved, they feel themselves to not be thin enough. It is however interesting to note that preoccupation with weight and body shape is not confined to anorectics but is frequently found in non-anorectic adolescents (Greenfield *et al.* 1987). This point brings us back to the notion of anorexia nervosa as a culture-bound syndrome (Swartz 1985) and the influence of media stereotypes referred to earlier.

Bulimia nervosa

Although bulimia nervosa has traditionally been thought of as a disorder of later adolescence and early adulthood, we felt it relevant to include it in this chapter for two reasons. First, bulimia often follows anorexia nervosa (Russell 1985) and food avoidance is replaced by over eating, and second, there is evidence to suggest that the incidence of bulimia may be increasing during adolescence and rates are now higher than during early adulthood (Connors and Johnson 1987). In addition, the incidence of bulimia is greater than anorexia. Shisslak *et al.* (1990), in a review of research, found incidence rates ranging from 0.4% to 16.2% in females and zero to 1.2% in males. Brown *et al.* (1989) found an incidence of 9%, and Muscari (1988) suggests that rates vary from 4.5% to 18%.

Typically the bulimic is white, female and middle class (Herzog 1988) and has a history of trying to diet without success. Some may be over-weight (Russell 1985). The bulimic will be obsessed with thoughts of food, and will binge varying quantities of food, particularly carbohy-drates (Conger 1988), on a regular basis. In some cases this will be daily and in others less frequently. Binging almost always takes place in secret (Russell 1985), and may be planned (Herzog 1982). Mitchell *et al.* (1981) found that binging was more likely to occur in the afternoon and eve-ning.

Following binges, bulimics may engage in various activities to rid their bodies of the food taken during the uncontrolled binge. These activities include manually induced vomiting, purging, amphetamine and diuretic use (Russell 1985), fasting and excessive exercise (Muscari 1988). These methods of getting rid of food may be undertaken in combination, or alone, but will bring a feeling of control back to the bulimic.

As with anorexia nervosa the precise causes of bulimia are unknown, although many predictions have been made which together form an interesting picture about the characteristics of the typical bulimic. Shisslak *et al.* (1990) reviewed the family background of bulimics and concluded that parental obesity, and a chaotic, undercontrolled and impulsive lifestyle were strongly associated with bulimic behaviour. Thus the bulimic has been brought up in an uncontrolled environment and they transfer this lack of control to eating patterns. They tend to be extravert, impulsive and moody. The mothers of bulimics are also somewhat typical, and tend to be 'home-makers' or involved in typically female occupations such as nursing. They have a tendency to drink heavily, have few friends and rely heavily on their daughters for emotional support (Muscari 1988). Bulimics report that binges are often triggered by their own alcohol use. Lacey (1985) found that bulimics tended to exhibit deficient emotional states, with bulimic behaviour acting as a stimulant to fulfil unmet need. Loneliness, boredom and depression would also frequently be cited as the trigger to binging. They also used bulimic behaviour to avoid feelings of guilt and anger. Body image disturbances are also frequently noted in bulimics. Muscari (1988) noted such disturbances which are also usual in anorectics. Muscari suggests that the difference between the two groups is that bulimics are aware of, and distressed by, their symptoms. In comparison to non-eating disordered controls, bulimics exhibit disordered body image, which includes misperceived weight status and body size, poor evaluation of fitness and health status, and unrealistically low assessments of physical appearance. Burckes-Miller and Black (1988) found similar body image distortions among college athletes – one third reported dramatic weight fluctuations relating to binging and fasting, and one seventh perceived themselves to be fat even though they were not.

A further interesting correlate with bulimia relates to sexuality and sexual experience. Russell (1985) notes that in bulimics who were previously anorectic, menstruation usually occurs or recurs as weight increases. Herzog (1988) suggests that bulimics are usually normal in terms of their sexuality. However Bulik *et al.* (1989) report high incidences of child sexual abuse in either the bulimic or female siblings. Other studies (see Lask and Bryant-Waugh 1992) have cited even higher incidences of abuse. Lask and Bryant-Waugh suggest, however, that the relationship between sexual abuse, family functioning and eating disorders remains uncertain, and that further research is needed to explore these complex variables. The causes of bulimia remain undefined.

The role of the nurse

The importance of understanding the complex background and nature of eating disorders cannot be overestimated. Nurses may be involved with eating-disordered adolescents in a variety of situations ranging from schools, clinics, children's wards, adolescent units, day units and in extreme cases, in-patient psychiatric units. Whilst the causes of disorders are as yet unfathomed, treatment regimes, particularly in relation to anorexia nervosa and bulimia, have changed with less emphasis being placed on medication in favour of enabling the young person and family to cope adaptively, rather than maladaptively with underlying problems

(Steinberg 1987). Adolescents, whether they present with obesity, anorexia nervosa or bulimia are likely to require support for long periods of time, and nurses have an important role to play, both independently and in collaboration with other members of the multidisciplinary team.

The goals of care

Eating disorders, as discussed in the preceding review, are symptoms rather than diseases. The primary aim of care should be to understand the perceptions of the disordered adolescent and the underlying pressures which precipitate the control of food intake. Assessing these pressures and perceptions may be a lengthy process, involving a variety of professionals. Nurses, however, are usually in the position of spending relatively lengthy amounts of time with the adolescent and family, particularly when the adolescent is admitted to hospital. Developing a good working relationship is an essential pre-requisite for care (Burns 1991) and the foundation for building trust and confidence. Approaches to care should be firm but consistent, and should reflect the views of the whole team (Steinberg 1987). The adolescent and the family should be aware of goals (Edelstein *et al.* 1989).

The essential differences in care between obese adolescents, anorectic and bulimic adolescents revolve around acceptance and recognition of fear. The obese adolescent usually has a strong desire to be thin, prompted by a lifetime of learning that thinness equals success. Although eating patterns may have deep and complex origins, they are essentially learned responses to specific cues (Conger 1991). That is not to say that obesity is easy to correct – a multi-million pound industry relies on the difficulty people have in losing weight. The point we are making is that because of cultural stereotypes, obese adolescents usually admit openly to their obesity and express a wish to be thinner.

This is not however the case with typical anorectics who have an intense fear of being fat, to the extent that they may deny their problems and refuse to co-operate with care which they know will lead to weight gain (Russell 1985). Fatness is seen as not only being equated with ugliness but also with being unloved and failing. Russell suggests that when setting goals with anorectics and their families, care should be taken to assess the anorectic's notion of a healthy weight. Again a consistent approach between carers is necessary. For example, reference to normative centile charts for weight may seem horrific to the anorectic, and throwaway comments such as 'we'll soon have you back to your old self' can destroy a tentative trust. Goals for the anorectic must therefore be realistic and attainable, and set in observable, measurable terms so that the adolescent knows exactly what is expected

(Muscari 1988). Danziger *et al.* (1988) suggest that a promise should be made to the anorectic that they will not become fat.

Bulimics also have an intense fear of fatness but are usually overtly distressed by their behaviour. That is not to say that anorectics are unaware. Palmer (1980) suggests:

'It is not that she (the anorectic) is immune to the miseries which self starvation brings, but rather that from her point of view they are outweighed by fear of change' (p 92).

What must be acknowledged in both anorectics and bulimics is that the disorders can act as identities for some adolescents and so the thought of gaining weight threatens to take away that identity. Fear of change is strong and may be a barrier to care.

Ultimately, the goals of care for eating-disordered adolescents must be then to attain a body weight which is within acceptable normative limits, to restore menstruation if the female adolescent has primary or secondary amenorrhoea, and to correct psychosocial dysfunctioning.

The process of care

A starting point for helping the adolescent with an eating disorder is to monitor patterns of eating and weight. Burns (1991), in her discussion of caring for bulimics, suggests the use of a food diary for the first few weeks of care. This can give insight into precipitating factors which can trigger binges. The use of a diary is also useful for the obese adolescent and, in the case of the anorectic, can help to identify thoughts and feelings about food. However, Burns suggests that the diary should not be a permanent feature of care and that the emphasis should be taken away from food rather than placed upon it. Muscari (1988), however, sees a diary which includes food intake and food related behaviour as an essential in adding a workable reality to disorders, which allows the adolescent to see progress being made. In the obese adolescent it is useful to use diary entries to identify stimuli which precede eating and to gain an understanding of the eating behaviour. Both stimuli and behaviour will ultimately need to be controlled (Graham 1985).

Regular weighing, which Danzinger *et al.* (1988) suggest should be daily for anorectics, is also an essential part of the process of care. Weighing sessions should not be taken lightly, as the adolescent, whether obese or underweight, will place great importance upon them. Nurses should be perceptive to the adolescent's feelings and should be wary of expressing subjective feelings towards weight gains and losses. An anorectic who has gained weight in excess of a goal, may feel out of control and positive reinforcement given by the nurse may be perceived by the anorectic as punishment in addition to the weight on the scales. The nurse should take cues from the adolescent, and reaffirm the promise that the gaining of a few kilos does not mean the young person will become fat whilst giving assurance that the gain in weight has improved appearance (Russell 1985). Danziger *et al.* (1988) also warn that nurses need to be aware of hidden objects which can add weight to the scales, and also of deliberate overhydration, which will also add temporary weight. Danziger *et al.* also suggest the use of privileges (such as eventually seeing friends) which can be introduced for co-operation.

Another important element of care relates to teaching. Muscari (1988) suggests that anorectics and bulimics may lack factual knowledge and have limited understanding of their disorder. This lack of knowledge may apply to obese adolescents also. Teaching is required which should highlight the interdependence between physiological and behavioural manifestations. Care must be taken, prior to teaching, to assess the adolescent's understanding. If teaching is not appropriate to cognitive ability it is unlikely to be effective (Taylor 1994). It is also useful to include the family in teaching sessions, but Muscari (1988) suggests that this should be done in a way which promotes the independence of the adolescent. Another important function of teaching is to explore the cultural pressures placed within society on thinness. Helping the adolescent to acknowledge that body shape does not guarantee happiness or success is a difficult but necessary function of helping the adolescent to understand disordered behaviour.

Other areas of care involve making constructive use of time. Whether the adolescent is in hospital or at home, boredom and loneliness are likely to exacerbate eating disorders. Encouraging the adolescent to draw up a schedule of activities is useful in identifying potential problem times, although Muscari (1988) suggests that all adolescents require what she describes as 'me time' – which is free time for themselves. The amount of supervision required by adolescents to ensure they conform to prescribed treatment regimes is also an important element of care, and one which requires balance. Russell (1985) suggests that the key to success with anorectics in hospital is a 'well-trained' nursing staff, who are confident in their ability to persuade the anorectic to eat the required amounts of food necessary to ensure a steady weight gain. The emphasis however should be placed upon the development of a positive relationship rather than on strict supervision. Whilst a certain amount of supervision will clearly be necessary it should not be oppressive and should nurture, rather than destroy, the nurse-adolescent relationship. Danziger *et al.* (1988), in their study of treating anorectics in day care, suggest that it is useful for parents to be involved in supervision, particularly after meals, to prevent vomiting and ritualistic exercise. This parental involvement allows parents to regain some of the control they usually feel they have lost.

Outcome

There is little research which discusses the long term effects of interventions with obese adolescents although behavioural modification was shown to have short term effects in a group of underprivileged obese adolescent girls (see Graham 1985). In terms of long term follow-up, Stunkard *et al.* (1980) found that behavioural techniques were more effective than interventions involving medication alone. In view of the large numbers of adolescents who are affected by this eating disorder, there is clearly a need for research with this group. We suggest that the paucity of recent study makes nurses ideally placed to undertake investigation in this field – particularly as they are very likely to come into contact with obese adolescents in almost every area of professional practice.

In terms of outcome for anorectics and bulimics, there is a slightly larger knowledge base. Bryant-Waugh *et al.* (1988), in a study of the long term outcomes of early onset eating disorders, found that several factors could influence long term success. They found high incidences of later eating problems, psychosocial and psychosexual dysfunction were more likely in adolescents who had an earlier onset age, who were depressed during their illness, who had disturbed family life, and who lived in one-parent families or in families where one or both parents had been married before. Overall Bryant-Waugh *et al.* suggest that the long term outlook is poor, 'psychiatric problems are common (in 50–70%) especially depression, obsessional behaviour, and social phobia' (p8). However, a study by Higgs *et al.* (1989) did not support these findings, and only correlated obsessionality at presentation, and premorbid height with poor outcome. An earlier study by Morgan and Russell (1975) found disturbed family relationships were predictive of poor outcome and, in contrast to Bryant-Waugh *et al.* (1988), found that late onset (rather than early onset) was correlated with poor outcome.

What remains clear is that for many adolescents with eating disorders, the outcome is less than favourable. Russell (1985) suggests that further longitudinal research is needed to ascertain the true extent of the effects of eating disorder, which may include infertility in anorectics, and long term psychosocial dysfunction.

Prevention

In Chapter 5 we have discussed health promotion strategies, and refer to eating disorders in the examples. However, this chapter would not be complete without discussing the prevention of these disorders, least of all because in a group of disorders with poor outcome, prevention is clearly important.

In view of the groups most at risk of developing serious disorders the most obvious place for prevention programmes is in school, although prevention programmes should not only be aimed at secondary school populations but at younger children whose attitudes and beliefs are being shaped by the world around them. We discussed in the section on obesity, for example, that children as young as 7 or 8 had already formed strong ideas about fatness. There is possibly an argument for starting prevention strategies even earlier, given the predictions relating to the role of the family in the development of eating disorders. Encouraging families to take meals together (Edelstein *et al.* 1989) and teaching young children about their dietary needs are two simple examples.

Prevention programmes in school should involve parents, teachers and pupils. Shisslak *et al.* (1990), in a pilot programme aimed at preventing eating disorders, suggest the use of formal presentations to staff, and to pupils, and a consultation component, whereby for a defined period of time each week, pupils or staff can seek individual advice. The formal programme suggested by Shisslak *et al.* involves covering the following topics:

- symptoms of eating disorders and their prevalence;
- psychological characteristics;
- medical complications;
- family characteristics;
- risk factors;
- treatment.

In addition to these topics, Shisslak *et al.* also suggest incorporating a 'self-esteem component', because of the association between low self-esteem and eating disorders. A further suggestion for curriculum content relates to body image and control. Burckes-Miller and Black (1988), in their study of eating behaviour among college athletes, concluded that students needed help in developing realistic body images, in controlling and mastering their eating behaviour, and in gaining a realistic perspective about food and weight.

Early detection

Working on an individual level with adolescents is a useful intervention which can be used as part of an overall programme of prevention, and also for the early detection of problems. School nurses developing student profiles are in an ideal position to undertake this role, and should be aware of the characteristics of disorders, particularly anorexia nervosa, because of the tendency to deny the disorder. Signs of noticeable weight loss, preoccupation with food or dieting, and a distorted body image are indicative of anorexia nervosa, but care should be taken not to jump to conclusions. Many pathophysiological conditions will, for example, cause weight loss. It is also possible that the anorectics and bulimics may seek advice for a related problem, such as menstrual irregularities or cold intolerance (Shisslak *et al.* 1990), gastrointestinal disturbances and sore throat, which are indicative of excessive vomiting and purging, palpitations and muscle spasms of the hands and feet, which relate to dehydration and electrolyte imbalances (Edelstein *et al.* 1989).

The implications for nurses

Clearly eating disorders are extremely complex. We know little about their causation but do know that many interacting variables probably contribute to their development. Nurses have a triple role in terms of these disorders. First, they are in an ideal position, particularly if they work in the field of health promotion, to explore with adolescents such issues as healthy nutrition, body image, self-esteem, and cultural and media opinion about body shape. Helping young people to feel comfortable and accepting of their bodies, as well as giving sensible advice about reaching and maintaining optimum body weight is of great importance. Second, nurses who work with adolescents, regardless of their specialist field of practice, should be aware of the potential for eating disorders among their clients and the need for the early detection of disorder. Finally, there are some nurses who may be involved in the therapy of adolescents who have diagnosed eating disorder. These nurses frequently face complex family situations, and young people who are confused and often extremely distressed. Interaction with these young people is unlikely to be transient, but will often last for many months if not years.

Our final comments in relation to eating disorders relate again to the lack of research by nurses in the UK into eating disorders. There is little evidence to suggest that eating disorders are becoming any less prevalent among adolescents in the UK, and yet the research base in relation to prevention, detection and nursing care is scarce. We would therefore urge nurses who work with adolescents to consider this an area of priority for future investigation.

References

Black, D. (1983) Obesity. *Journal of the Royal College of Physicians of London*, 17: 5–65.

Bouchard, C. *et al.* (1990) The response to long-term overfeeding in identical twins. *New England Journal of Medicine*, 322: 1477–1482.

Brown, T.A., Cash, T.F. and Lewis, R.J. (1989) Body image disturbances in adolescent female binge-purgers: a brief report of the results of a national survey in the USA. *Journal of Child Psychology and Psychiatry*, 30(4): 605–613.

Bruch, H. (1982) Anorexia nervosa: therapy and theory. *American Journal of Psychiatry*, 139(12): 1531–1538.

Bryant-Waugh, R., Knibbs, J., Fosson, A., Kaminski, Z. and Lask, B. (1988) Long term follow up of patients with early onset anorexia nervosa. *Archives of Disease in Childhood*, 63: 5–9.

Bulik, C., Sullivan, P. and Rorty, M. (1989) Childhood sexual abuse in women with bulimia. *Journal of Clinical Psychiatry*, 50: 229–233.

Burckes-Miller, M.E. and Black, D.R. (1988) Behaviours and attitudes associated with eating disorders: perceptions of college athletes about food and weight. *Health Education Research*, 3(2): 203–208.

Burns, J.S. (1991) Anorexia bulimia. In: *Child Care: Some Nursing Perspectives.* (Ed. A. Glasper) Wolfe, London.

Conger, J.J. (1988) Hostages to fortune: youth, values and the public interest. *American Psychologist*, 43: 291–300.

Conger, J.J. (1991) *Adolescence and Youth: Psychological Development in a Changing World*, 4th edn. Harper and Row, New York.

Connors, M. and Johnson, C. (1987) Epidemiology of bulimia and bulimic behaviors. *Addictive Behaviors*, 12: 165–179.

Crisp, A.H. (1980) *Anorexia Nervosa: Let Me Be.* Academic Press, London.

Danziger, Y., Carcl, C., Varsano, I., Tyano, S and Mimouni, M. (1988) Parental involvement in the treatment of patients with anorexia nervosa in a pediatric day-care unit. *Pediatrics*, 81(1): 159–162.

Department of Health and Social Security (1984) *Report of the Panel on Diet in Relation to Cardiovascular Disease.* HMSO, London.

Dietz, W.H. (1990) You are what you eat – what you eat is what you are. *Journal of Adolescent Health Care*, 11: 76–81.

Edelstein, C.K., Haskew, P. and Kramer, J.P. (1989) Early clues to anorexia and bulimia. *Patient Care*, 23(13): 155–158, 161, 164, 167–168, 175.

Eisele, J., Hertsgaard, D. and Light, H. (1986) Factors related to eating disorders in young adolescent girls. *Adolescence*, 21: 283–290.

Fisher, J. (1990) What our children are eating: a report on the diets of 14–16 years old school children in the Thames Valley. *Health at School*, 5(5): 150–154.

Fontaine, K.L. (1991) The conspiracy of culture: women's issues in body size. *Nursing Clinics of North America*, 26(3): 669–676.

Garner, D.M. and Garfinkel, P.E. (1980) Sociocultural factors in the development of anorexia nervosa. *Psychological Medicine*, 10: 647–656.

Gowers, S.G., Crisp, A.H., Joughlin, N. and Bhat, A. (1991) Premenstrual anorexia nervosa. *Journal of Child Psychology and Psychiatry*, 32(3): 515–524.

Graham, P.J. (1985) Psychosomatic relationships. In: *Child and Adolescent Psychiatry*. (Ed. M. Rutter and L. Hersov) Blackwell Scientific Publications, Oxford.

Greenfield, D., Quinlan, D.M., Harding, P., Glass, E. and Bliss, A. (1987) Eating behaviour in an adolescent population. *International Journal of Eating Disorders*, 6: 99–112.

Hawk, L. and Brook, C. (1979) Family resemblances of height, weight and body fatness. *Archives of Disease in Childhood*, 54: 877–879.

Health Education Council (1983) *National Advisory Committee in Nutrition Education (NACNE): Proposals for Nutrition Guidelines for Health Education in Britain.* HEC, London.

Herzog, D.B. (1982) Bulimia: the secretive syndrome. *Psychosomatics*, 23: 481–487.

Herzog, D.B. and Copeland, P.M. (1985) Eating disorders. *New England Journal of Medicine*, 313(5): 295–303.

Herzog, D.B. (1988) Eating disorders. In: *The New Harvard Guide to Psychiatry*. (Ed. A.M. Nicholi) Harvard University Press, Cambridge, Mass.

Higgs, J.F., Goodyer, I.M. and Birch, J. (1989) Anorexia nervosa and food avoidance emotional disorder. *Archives of Disease in Childhood*, 64: 346–351.

Holland, A.J., Hall, A., Murray, R., Russell, G.F.M. and Crisp, A.H. (1984) Anorexia nervosa: a study of 34 twin pairs and one set of triplets. *British Journal of Psychiatry*, 145: 414–419.

Hsu, L.K.G. (1990) *Eating Disorders*. Guildford Press, New York.

Johnson-Sabine, E., Wood, K., Patton, G., Mann, A. and Wakeling, A. (1988) Abnormal eating attitudes in London schoolgirls – a prospective epidemiological study: factors associated with abnormal response on screening questionnaires. *Psychological Medicine*, 18: 615–622.

Kalucy, R. (1976) Obesity: an attempt to find a common ground among some of the biological, psychological and sociological phenomena of the obesity/overeating syndrome. In: *Modern Trends in Psychosomatic Medicine, 3*. (Ed. O. Hill) Butterworths, London.

Kaplan, K.A. and Wadden, T.A. (1986) Childhood obesity and self-esteem. *Journal of Paediatrics*, 109: 367–370.

King, M.B. (1989) Eating disorders in a general practice population: prevalence, characteristics and follow-up at 12 and 18 months. *Psychological Medicine*. Monograph Supplement No 14.

Lacey, J.H. (1985) Time limited individual and group treatment for bulimia. In: *Handbook of Psychotherapy for Anorexia Nervosa and Bulimia*. (Eds D.M. Garner and P.S. Garfinkel) Guilford Press, London.

Larson, R. and Johnson, C. (1982) Anorexia nervosa in context of daily living. *Journal of Youth and Adolescence*, 10: 455–471.

Lask, B. and Bryant-Waugh, R. (1992) Early-onset anorexia nervosa and related eating disorders. *Journal of Child Psychology and Psychiatry*, 33(1): 281–300.

Ledoux, S., Choquet, M and Flament, M. (1991) Eating disorders among adolescents in an unsettled French population. *International Journal of Eating Disorders*, 10: 81–89.

Love, C.C. and Seaton, H. (1991) Eating disorders: highlights of nursing assessment and therapeutics. *Nursing Clinics of North America*, 26(3): 677–697.

McNamara, D.J. (1986) Diet and heart disease: mass interventions or individualised treatments? In: *A Diet of Reason*. (Ed. D. Anderson) Social Affairs Unit, London.

Mitchell, J.E., Pyle, R.L. and Eckert, E.D. (1981) Frequency and duration of binge-eating episodes in patients with bulimia. *American Journal of Psychiatry*, 141: 835–836.

Morgan, H.G. and Russell, G.F.M. (1975) Value of family background and clinical features as predictors of long-term outcome in anorexia nervosa: four year follow-up study of 41 patients. *Psychological Medicine*, 5: 355–371.

Muscari, M. (1988) Effective nursing strategies for adolescents with anorexia nervosa and bulimia nervosa. *Pediatric Nursing*, 14(6): 475–482.

Palmer, R.L. (1980) *Anorexia Nervosa*. Penguin, Harmondsworth.

Passmore, R. (1986) Obesity and plumpness which needs no diet. In: *A Diet of Reason*. (Ed. D. Anderson) Social Affairs Unit, London.

Russell, G.F.M. (1985) Anorexia and bulimia nervosa. In: *Child and Adolescent Psychiatry*, 2nd edn. (Eds M. Rutter and L. Hersov) Blackwell Scientific Publications, Oxford.

Shisslak, C.M., Crago, M. and Neal, M. (1990) Prevention of eating disorders among adolescents. *American Journal of Health Promotion*, 5(2): 100–106.

Showalter, E. (1987) *The Female Malady: Women, Madness and English Culture*. Virago, London.

Slade, R. (1984) *Anorexia Nervosa Reference Book*. Harper and Row, London.

Stark, O., Atkins, E., Wolff, O.H. and Douglas, J.W.B. (1981) Longitudinal study of obesity in the National Survey of Health and Development. *British Medical Journal*, 283: 13–17.

Steinberg, D. (1987) *Basic Adolescent Psychiatry*. Blackwell Scientific Publications, Oxford.

Streigel-Moore, R.H., Silberstein, L.R. and Rodin, J. (1986) Towards an understanding of risk factors for bulimia. *American Psychologist*, 41: 246–263.

Strober, M., Lampert, C., Morrell, W., Burroughs, J. and Jacobs, C. (1990) A controlled family study of anorexia nervosa. *International Journal of Eating Disorders*, 9: 239–253.

Stunkard, A.J. and Burt, V. (1967) Obesity and body image: age at onset of disturbances in the body image. *American Journal of Psychiatry*, 123: 1443–1447.

Stunkard, A.J., Craighead, L.W. and O'Brien, R. (1980) Controlled trial of behavioural therapy, pharmacotherapy and their combination in the treatment of obesity. *Lancet*, ii: 1045–1047.

Stunkard, A.J. (1985) Obesity. In: *Comprehensive Textbook of Psychiatry*, 4th edn. (Eds H.I. Kaplan and B.J. Sadock) Williams and Wilkins, Baltimore.

Stunkard, A.J., Harris, J.R., Pederson, N.L. and McClearn, G.E. (1990) The body-mass index of twins who have been reared apart. *New England Journal of Medicine*, 322: 1483–1487.

Swartz, L. (1985) Anorexia nervosa as a culture-bound syndrome. *Social Science Medicine*, 20(7): 725–730.

Swift, W.J., Bushness, N.J., Hanson, P. and Logemann, T. (1986) Self-concept in adolescent anorexics. *Journal of the American Academy of Child Psychiatry*, 25(6): 826–835.

Tanner, J.M. and Whitehouse, R.H. (1975) Revised standards for triceps and subcapsular skinfolds in British children. *Archives of Disease in Childhood*, 41: 454–471.

Taylor, J. (1994) The well and sick adolescent. In: *Health Promotion and Patient Education*. (Ed. P. Webb) Chapman and Hall, London.

Tobias, A.L. and Gordon, J.B. (1980) Social consequences of obesity. *Journal of the American Dietetic Association*, 76: 338–342.

Further reading

Hsu, L.K.G. (1990) *Eating Disorders*. Guilford Press, New York.
This very readable book explores the many complex aspects of eating disorders and factors which may contribute to their development.

Garner, D.M. and Garfinkel, P.E. (eds) (1985) *Handbook of Psychotherapy for Anorexia Nervosa and Bulimia*. Guilford Press, London.
This book explores various aspects of therapy and although it is old it is well worth reading.

Chapter 8

Human Immunodeficiency Virus and Acquired Immunodeficiency Syndrome in Adolescence

Over the last decade knowledge about the human immunodeficiency virus (HIV) and the acquired immunodeficiency syndrome (AIDS) has increased dramatically. We are constantly bombarded with a plethora of information, from both lay and professional sources. Some of the information we receive is contradictory, some is sensationalist and some merely perpetuates the myths which surround HIV and AIDS. This chapter aims to explore the issue of HIV and AIDS during adolescence with particular emphasis on how nurses can provide sensitive and competent health promotion and care. We start by discussing how adolescents may become HIV positive and how this can impact upon adolescent development.

Adolescents at risk

It is not currently possible to accurately predict how many adolescents in the UK are HIV positive. As far as we are aware there have been no studies which have randomly tested large groups of adolescents in order to ascertain prevalence. What is clear however is that adolescents are at risk for a number of reasons, not least because of the increased incidence of risk-taking behaviour during this period. Furthermore a study among adolescents in the USA (Burke *et al.* 1990) found a rate of HIV infection of 0.35 per 1000 males and 0.32 per 1000 females. Whilst this study involved screening army recruits (over one million of them), and cannot be generalized to British adolescents, it does suggest that the virus may now be prevalent among young people.

There are a number of ways in which adolescents have, and could, become HIV positive – not all of which relate to adolescent behaviour. There are also some modes of transmission which are no longer problematic, for example infection through the receipt of infected factor VIII. We have however included these modes of transmission in this discussion not least because, whilst the threat of infection through certain mediums may have ceased, there remain groups of young people who were infected through medical intervention, and who may well come into contact with the health services.

Blood and blood products

The first description of AIDS in a child was in 1982 (see Prose 1990). The child was thought to have acquired the infection after receiving a blood transfusion. Over the next few years it was identified that infection could not only be acquired through receiving infected blood, but also through the receipt of blood products, infected organs and bone marrow.

Factor VIII, a vital clotting component of blood, is perhaps one of the saddest examples of how children (and indeed adults) became infected with the virus through the receipt of infected blood products. The administration of factor VIII had promised to ease the symptoms of many children and adults with haemophilia by providing the missing component within their own blood clotting mechanisms. However, by the mid 1980s it was apparent that blood for transfusion, and for the manufacture of blood products such as factor VIII, had been contaminated with HIV. Since 1986 factor VIII has been treated to inactivate the virus, however, a large number of haemophiliacs had already been infected in this way. Schroeder (1993) reports that, by the end of 1992, 1235 people with haemophilia had tested HIV positive. Many have unfortunately already died. It is also perhaps worth mentioning that treating blood and blood products is expensive and in some developing countries and parts of Eastern Europe does not take place. Transmission through this route is therefore still a problem in some parts of the world (Moriasy and Thomas 1990).

Sexual transmission

The first reported incidence of AIDS was among homosexual young men in the USA and in the early 1980s the virus was thought to be exclusive to homosexual men. It became known colloquially as the 'gay plague'. However, it soon became clear that the virus could be transmitted through heterosexual intercourse, and more recent projections suggest that heterosexual intercourse is the most frequent source of transmission (Jackson 1991).

In Chapter 3 we have already discussed the sexual development of adolescents, and there is a growing body of knowledge to suggest that adolescents are at risk through sexual behaviour (Woodcock *et al.* 1992; Mellanby *et al.* 1993). In spite of large-scale national campaigns which promote safer sex, many adolescents continue to put themselves at risk through unprotected homosexual and heterosexual intercourse. The initial targetting of gay men led to a greater awareness of the need for safer sex. The effect of this targetting was, however, according to Jackson (1991) to the detriment of women who did not perceive themselves as being at risk. Local and national campaigns have attempted to redress the balance and have targetted heterosexual people. However, a similar situation may now be occurring among new young gay men (Linehan 1993) who are reaching sexual maturity and who do not remember the original health promotion campaigns. These young men are particularly at risk for two reasons. First because Clause 28 of the 1988 Local Government Bill prohibits maintained schools from teaching about the acceptability of homosexuality (see Patrick 1988). Secondly, homosexual intercourse is illegal in young men under the age of 18 years which may discourage them from seeking help and advice about safer sex or sexual health problems from statutory services. Linehan (1993) suggests that these groups need to be targetted consistently in order to reach young people who are becoming sexually active. Females and sex workers (both male and female) are particularly at risk because safer sex relies on male partners co-operation (Jackson 1991: Reid 1993). Mangan (1993) in a report of the Idaho Project, which is a service for adolescents and young men who are sex workers, suggests that their risk of contracting HIV is high because traditionally they have not practised safer sex and their clients are often unwilling to use condoms. Mangan suggests that it is important for these young men to learn to be assertive and to negotiate the use of protection.

It is not only adolescents who voluntarily consent to sexual intercourse who are at risk of becoming infected with HIV. Sexual abuse of children and adolescents was highlighted by the *Butler-Sloss Report* (1988) which focused on the potential misdiagnosis of sexual abuse, but at the same time brought to the attention of professionals the probability that sexual abuse of children and adolescents was not an isolated problem. Since the report a great deal of further investigation has taken place which has highlighted the potential scale of the problem (Hobbs and Wynne 1990). Adolescents who are sexually abused are clearly at risk of HIV infection and health professionals should be aware of this potential. This awareness should extend to both female and male rape victims who, after their initial trauma, must face the possibility that they may have been infected. Rape survivors should be carefully counselled by trained counsellors and offered HIV testing.

Intravenous drug users

In Chapter 9 we discuss substance abuse and some of the epidemiological data relating to intravenous drug use. Research which correlates HIV infection and intravenous drug use in adolescents is, as yet, limited – although increased knowledge about the natural history of HIV and AIDS suggests that many adults who are HIV positive and who have AIDS through drug use probably became infected during adolescence (Brettle and Nelles 1985). The practice of sharing needles and other equipment for 'main-lining' carries with it the risk of contracting HIV. Studies suggest that, whilst intravenous drug use among adolescents is low when compared with other forms of substance abuse, as many as 1% of adolescents may use intravenous drugs (Health Education Authority 1992; Advisory Council on the Misuse of Drugs 1993). Clearly, health promotion in relation to drug abuse is an important strategy in the prevention of HIV infection.

Vertical transmission

In 1983 the Centers for Communicable Diseases in the USA identified that some of the children born to HIV positive mothers were infected with the virus. The risk of a baby becoming infected through vertical transmission is thought to be around 13% (Claxton 1993). This is lower than earlier estimates derived from research in Europe and the United States which estimated transmission rates of between 24 and 35% (see Husson *et al.* 1990). Despite revised transmission rates, vertical transmission is likely in future to be the more usual mode of infection among children, particularly as children with haemophilia in the developed world should no longer be at risk.

Many of the children born to infected mothers who contracted the virus have died. The course of HIV in children is different from adults and estimates suggest that 25% of infected children will develop AIDS during the first year of life and a staggering 80% by the end of the fourth year of life (WHO cited in Chin 1990). There are however young adolescents who became infected through vertical transmission who remain well, and whilst they number few at present, it can be anticipated that a growing number of adolescents will have become HIV positive through infection *in utero* or through infected breast milk. These young people clearly face a multitude of psychological and social problems, which we will discuss later. There is also the obvious possibility that either one or both parents may be ill or will have died. Mothers, by virtue of having transmitted the virus vertically, must be HIV positive, and fathers may have become infected also. Vertical transmission is also a potential problem for HIV positive adolescents who become pregnant and a growing number of young people are facing the dilemma of remaining childless or to risk passing the virus on to negative partners and children.

Promoting healthy behaviours

As we have discussed above adolescents are at risk of contracting HIV for a number of reasons and one of the important areas where nurses can help adolescents relates to the promotion of healthy behaviours. We have discussed the principles of health promotion in Chapter 5 but now relate these principles specifically to risk-taking behaviour and HIV.

Promoting sexual health

The sexual health of young people has been highlighted as a key target in the Government's *Health of the Nation* report (DoH 1992), in recognition of the potential risks to young people in terms of pregnancy and sexually transmitted diseases including HIV and AIDS. Promoting safer sexual practices is clearly one part of the strategy, as is encouraging young people to think very carefully before they become sexually active. There is evidence that extending the age at which young people become sexually active could certainly affect risk taking behaviour. Mellanby *et al.* (1993) in a large study of 15 and 16 year old show that there is a correlation between age of first sexual intercourse and risk-taking behaviour. Young people who start sexual relationships before the age of 16 years are less likely to practice safer sex than those who first have sexual intercourse after the age of 16 years.

A second study (Dilorio *et al.* 1993) has suggested that, whilst adolescents may have a high standard of knowledge about the transmission of HIV, there are gaps in their knowledge concerning safer sex practices such as the use of spermicide and the use of certain types of condom. Dockrell and Joffe (1992) also found in their study that 'there is often a mismatch between individuals' interpretation of safer sex and that intended by the institution which transmits the message' (p 509). Dockrell and Joffe suggest that some young people have difficulty in accepting the safer sex message. They found that, whilst most young people in their research claimed to practice safer sex, they did not *always* do so, particularly when they had sexual intercourse with a new partner. Part of the problem appears to be an inability for young people to view themselves as being at risk. Dockrell and Joffe found that there were two groups of individuals who saw themselves as immune. The first group were those who did not see HIV/AIDS as their problem and so did not practice safer sex, and the second group were those who practised safer sex and therefore saw themselves as being no longer at risk. Many of the young people interviewed felt they could intuitively identify if a partner was HIV positive, which in view of the national campaigns which clearly advertise that it is impossible to know, is a worrying finding. The young people in this study also felt that if they *knew* their partner they were safe. On further probing however, the adolescents definitions of knowing, ranged from being acquainted for years to being acquainted for only hours.

Health promotion in schools is clearly a vital part of encouraging young people to avoid risk-taking behaviours. However, the whole issue of sex education in schools is problematic. Under the Education Act 1986, power to decide if, and in what form, sex education should take place was vested in school governors and then parents. A recent circular (see Cohen 1994) has made sex education compulsory from September 1994 but prohibits teachers from giving individual advice about contraception without parental consent. We welcome the compulsory teaching of sex education. In a review of the current state of sex education in schools, Tattam (1993) reports that as many as 50% of schools prior to the 1994 circular did not encourage instruction on sexual health, and that sex education in schools was being jeopardized by school governors. Jackson (1991) suggested that the number of schools 'opting out' of Local Authority Control was potentially increasing this problem, as opted out schools do have to comply with Local Authority policy, if such a policy existed. As mentioned previously, schools are also prohibited from teaching about homosexuality, despite estimates that 10% of pupils are either lesbian or gay (Patrick 1988). This presents a second difficulty for health promoters in schools, as a significant proportion of young people may feel that education about safer sex is not relevant to them specifically.

Where schools do run programmes on sexual health it is important that adolescents receive accurate information which is both age and culture sensitive. The important messages which must reach young people is that early intercourse and multiple partners are correlated not only with an increased risk of HIV infection, but also with other medical risks such as cervical cancer (Curtis *et al.* 1989). It is also important to educate young people in the practice of safer sex. Woodcock *et al.* (1992) in their study of sex education found that many young people had not been educated in the use of contraception, particularly in relation to the safe use of condoms. Others said that sex education had come too late for them. One adolescent girl had already become pregnant and had a termination by the time contraception was covered in school. Her comment of 'Oh great, now you tell me' is particularly poignant.

It is suggested that with the falling age of puberty and the rise in adolescent pregnancies it is appropriate for sex education to commence in primary school (Jackson 1991) although if this does take place it is important that teachers and nurses are trained to undertake such education. At whatever age health education takes place, it must be both relevant and sensitive to the adolescent's age and cognitive ability (Taylor 1994). Schools should investigate effective ways of delivering health promotion and should evaluate the efficacy of education strategies.

An example of an experimental approach to sexual health promotion is highlighted by Jackson (1991) who reports on a strategy at Luton sixth form college, where each year ten students of mixed race, gender and academic ability are trained in HIV/AIDS awareness. These young people then run workshops for their peers which are proving to be highly successful as peer group training appears to break down barriers and promote more open discussion.

Safer drug use

Whilst it is clearly not appropriate to promote drug use, there will always be young people who misuse substances as a way of coping with their lives. Fortunately, as mentioned above, the numbers of young people who inject drugs is small. However, approximately 1% of adolescents may inject drugs which represents a significant number of young people who may be at risk of contracting HIV infection. Due to the great interest in HIV infection and associated drug misuse the development of 'harm minimization strategies' have enabled effective intervention among adolescent drug users (Farrell and Strang 1991). Such harm minimization includes informing young people about safer syringe cleaning techniques, needle exchange programmes and first aid resuscitation as well as providing information and support for drug rehabilitation.

There are also clear links between substance abuse and high risk sexual activity (Robertson and Plant 1988), and health promoters need to be aware of these links. Suggesting that one partner remain 'straight' enough to ensure that safer sex (rather than unsafe sex) takes place may well fall on deaf ears, and assumes that sex is always a planned activity, which clearly it is not. It is certainly a difficult problem and health promoters can only encourage drug users to be prepared for safer sex and hope that their advice is heeded.

HIV and adolescent development

Young people who are HIV positive face an uncertain future with varying amounts of social support. In Chapter 4 we discuss the tasks of adolescence and it is perhaps useful to use those tasks as a framework for discussing the implications of HIV. The tasks were:

● adjusting to a rapidly changing physique and sexual development;

- achieving a sense of independence from parents;
- acquiring the social skills of a young adult;
- developing the necessary academic and vocational skills;
- developing a sense of oneself as a worthwhile person;
- achieving an internalized set of guiding norms and values.

Adolescents who are HIV positive may require a great deal of help in approaching and working through some of these important tasks. Young people who are HIV positive face, for example, difficult decisions in relation to sexual activity and their future as parents. Schroeder (1993), in a discussion of the needs of the female partners of adolescents with haemophilia, cites Lee, Director of the Haemophilia Centre at the Royal Free Hospital in London:

'For teenagers and their girlfriends, the biggest problem is that boys may not declare that they are people with haemophilia who are also HIV positive. We try to encourage them to be responsible, but it is difficult, as there is little incentive for them to disclose the information to their female partners' (p36).

The decision as to whether to have children is one that may be faced during adolescence, and even when such decisions occur much later, adolescents who are HIV positive have to live with the possibility that they may never have children, or that their children may become infected through vertical transmission. Encouraging reports from the Royal Free Hospital (in Schroeder 1993) show that of the 14 couples where the father had both haemophilia and was HIV positive, who had planned to have a baby, one mother had become infected, but none of the babies. Clearly, the numbers involved are too small to generalize at present but such data can give hope to adolescents. What is important is that adolescents who are HIV positive need skilful counselling before they decide to have a child, particularly in relation to the future, but also in relation to putting their partners at the least risk possible during conception.

A second task of adolescence which may be difficult for young people who are HIV positive relates to vocational choice. It is sad that the health professions, which are committed to equal opportunity, may be difficult career choices for adolescents. For example, one young man who wished to become a nurse claims he was unable to fulfil his chosen vocation because of his HIV status (Carlisle 1993a). Similarly, medicine and dentistry may be prohibited careers because of the students inability to participate in mandatory elements of courses (see DoH 1993).

Who needs to know?

In the 1980s there was a certain amount of widespread panic about HIV and AIDS which was partially fuelled by media reporting but also by public (and professional) ignorance. Some HIV positive individuals were (and still are) refused life insurance or mortgages, and refused entry to certain countries.

There were also reports of parents, on finding out that an HIV positive child was attending school, who kept their own children at home rather than let them come into contact with HIV (Stevens *et al.* 1993). Mackie (cited in Francis 1993) also reported that some mothers believed that their children could contract the virus by sitting next to an HIV positive child. This was in spite of widespread reassurance that the virus could not be transmitted through normal social contact. Parents and adolescents may be reluctant to inform schools of their HIV status because of the fear of isolation and the potential for prejudice. Schools should in any case take precautions when dealing with body fluids regardless of known risk.

Clearly, as with all patients and clients, nurses in order to comply with the UKCC's *Code of Professional Conduct* (1992) must afford patients confidentiality and must not divulge any information without the informed consent of the client. Mayho (interviewed by Carlisle 1993b) claims that some nurses 'seem to leave confidentiality at the workplace' which is obviously unacceptable practice. Where adolescents are HIV positive, we believe that this consent should come from the adolescent as well as the parents, and where they disagree about who should be told, every attempt should be made to refer both the adolescent and the parents to a trained counsellor who can explore with them all the implications of informing others about HIV status.

As we have discussed above there is also the issue of young health workers who may be HIV positive. The public panic of the 1980s still persists to a certain extent, particularly in relation to health workers. Some doctors, for example, have found themselves at the centre of a great deal of unwanted attention when their HIV status has been highlighted. There have been similar instances involving nurses. Mayho (in Carlisle 1993b) a young male ex-student nurse who probably contracted HIV from his first lover when he was 16 years old, claims he was forced to 'resign' after reporting his HIV status to the hospital's occupational health department.

Helping HIV positive adolescents and their families

Nurses who are in contact with HIV positive adolescents and their families are clearly in a position to be able to offer support and guidance, as well as ensuring that appropriate counselling is offered, preferably from a clinical psychologist. At present adolescents who are HIV positive are likely to come from families where there are other members who are infected, or where there is a family history of haemophilia. Family centred care is therefore important and nurses must ensure that they are absolutely up-to-date in terms of their knowledge bases. It is important that nurses address their own potential prejudices about sexuality and HIV/AIDS, which may be a barrier to effective care.

The Mildmay Mission Hospital is an example of a service which is aiming to address the dearth of family centred services for people with HIV and AIDS. The hospital offers respite care for affected individuals and their families, and focuses not only on physical needs, but also on psychosocial and spiritual care which is important as AIDS can be a particularly isolating illness (Dart and Taylor 1993). Another example of a specialist service is the Griffin project which is an HIV unit for drug users, who Cooper (1992) suggests need space and time to plan their lives effectively.

The implications for nurses

The implication for nurses who are involved in HIV prevention or in caring for young people who are HIV positive are extremely complex. Nurses are not immune to the media attention which has focused on HIV and AIDS and may feel frightened and vulnerable when they first become involved in caring for adolescents who are HIV positive. It is however important that nurses do not fail in their duty to those who need their care.

A duty to care

HIV positive adolescents and their families have a right to receive high standards of care and nurses have a duty to participate in that care. In 1990 the UKCC heard its first case involving a nurse who refused to care for an HIV positive patient. The nurse was struck off the UKCC professional register (*Nursing Times* 1990). The clear message is that nurses do not have the right to pick and choose the patients they care for.

Whilst nurses have a duty to care for patients regardless of their HIV status, such care should also be anti-discriminatory. The Royal College of Nursing (RCN) ran a series of workshops (see Rose and Platzer 1993) and participants reported negative behaviour by nurses in relation to the care of lesbians and gay men. Assumptions were made about their lifestyles and examples of nurses assuming that homosexuality equalled HIV positive status were given. One patient's charts were visibly labelled 'high risk' simply because he was gay. Similar examples were highlighted in a study of HIV positive patients in North Thames (Association of London Authorities/North East Thames Regional Health Authority 1992). Patients in intensive care units reported having notes labelled with 'high risk' and 'AIDS', which were visible to visitors and other patients. Nurses in this study were criticized for their attitude and lack of respect.

Anti-discriminatory practices were also noted by Laurent (1993) in a discussion of male rape victims, who were assumed by staff to be 'kinky gays'. Laurent suggests that nurses need to be aware of, and address their own potential and actual prejudices.

Providing care

To conclude this chapter on HIV and AIDS in adolescence we felt it might be useful to reiterate the views of the late Richard Wells in relation to caring for HIV positive patients and clients. He wrote (Wells 1988) that caring for HIV positive clients will challenge nurses but that they should respond by providing:

● meaningful acute care in the hospital and community setting;
● continuing care;
● leaving or returning control to the patient;
● support of those close to the patient;
● confidentiality;
● patient advocacy.

The attitude and behaviour of nurses then who are in a position where they may be interacting with adolescents and their families who are HIV positive can make an immense difference to those who they are caring for. Acknowledging that HIV and AIDS do not only affect individuals but affect all those who are involved with the HIV positive individual is vital. HIV and AIDS, as relatively new 'conditions', have had an unfortunate beginning involving a great deal of prejudice, stereotyping and fear. Nurses can help their clients, families and others to overcome their negative feelings and think positively about the future.

References

Advisory Council on the Misuse of Drugs (1993) *Drug Education in Schools.* HMSO, London.

Association of London Health Authorities in conjunction with North East Thames Regional Health Authority (1992) *A Need to Listen*. London.

Burke, D.S., Brundage, J.F., Goldenbaum, H., Gardner, L., Peterson, M., Visintirie, R. and Redfield, R.R. (1990) Human immunodeficiency virus infections in teenagers: seroprevalence among applicants for US military service. *Journal of the American Medical Association*, 263: 2074–2077.

Brettle, R. and Nelles, B. (1988) Special problems of injecting drug-misusers. In: *AIDS and HIV Infection: the Wider Perspective. British Medical Bulletin*, 44(1): 149–160.

Butler-Sloss, E. (1988) *Report of the Inquiry into Child Abuse in Cleveland 1987*. HMSO, London.

Carlisle, D. (1993a) Broken promise. *Nursing Times*, 89(19): 22.

Carlisle, D. (1993b) Professional help. *Nursing Times*, 89(48): 24–26.

Chin, J. (1990) Epidemiology: current and future dimensions of the HIV/AIDS pandemic in women and children. *Lancet*, 336: 221–224.

Claxton, R. (1993) *HIV and AIDS: Information about Mothers and Children with HIV Infection*. Terence Higgins Trust, London.

Cohen, P. (1994) The role of the school nurse in providing sex education. *Nursing Times*, 90(23): 36–38.

Cooper, C. (1992) Time to think. *Community Care*, 941: 25.

Curtis, H., Lawrence, C. and Tripp, J. (1989) Teenage sexuality: implications for controlling AIDS. *Archives of Disease in Childhood*, 64: 1240–1245.

Dart, S. and Taylor, E. (1993) Talking it through. *Nursing Times*, 89(16): 50–52.

Department of Health (1992) *Health of the Nation*. HMSO, London.

Department of Health (1993) *AIDS/HIV – Infected Health-Care Workers: Guidance on the Management of Infected Health-Care Workers*. DoH, London.

Dilorio, C., Parsons, M. and Lehr, S. (1993) Knowledge of AIDS and safer sex practices among college freshmen. *Public Health Nursing*, 10(3): 159–165.

Dockrell, J. and Joffe, H. (1992) Methodological issues involved in the study of young people and HIV/AIDS: a social psychological view. *Health Education Research*, 7(H): 509–516.

Farrell, M. and Strang, J. (1991) Substance use and misuse in childhood and adolescence. *Journal of Child Psychology and Psychiatry*, 32(1): 109–128.

Francis, J. (1993) A jolt in the right direction. *Community Care*, 955: 9.

Health Education Authority (1992) *Tomorrow's Young Adults*. HEA, London.

Hobbs, C.J. and Wynne, J.M. (1990) The sexually abused battered child. *Archives of Disease in Childhood*, 65: 423–427.

Husson, R.N., Corneau, A. and Hoff, R. (1990) Diagnosis of human immunodeficiency virus in infants and children. *Paediatrics*, 86(1): 1–9.

Jackson, C. (1991) Getting the message across. *Health Visitor*, 64(7): 212–213.

Laurent, C. (1993) Male rape. *Nursing Times*, 89(6): 18–19.

Linehan, T. (1993) Barred from safe sex. *Nursing Times*, 89(12): 16–17.

Mangan, P. (1993) Men at work. *Nursing Times*, 89(48): 29–30

Mellanby, A., Phelps, F. and Tripp, J.H. (1993) Teenagers, sex and risk taking. *British Medical Journal*, 307(6895): 25.

Moriasy, J. and Thomas, L. (1990) *Triple Jeopardy – Women and AIDS*. Panos Books.

Nursing Times News (1990) Nurse struck off for refusal to treat AIDS. *Nursing Times*, 86(51): 5.

Patrick, P. (1988) Sex education, homosexuality and the law. *Health at School*, 3(7): 201–202.

Prose, N. (1990) HIV infection in children. *Journal of the American Academy of Dermatology*, 22: 1223–1231.

Reid, T. (1993) Positive thinking. *Nursing Times*, 89(48): 26–28.

Robertson, J.A. and Plant, M.A. (1988) Alcohol, sex and risks of HIV infection. *Drug and Alcohol Dependence*, 22: 75–78.

Rose, P. and Platzer, H. (1993) Confronting prejudice. *Nursing Times*, 89(31): 52–54.

Schroeder, J. (1993) Partners in need. *Nursing Times*, 89(4): 36–39.

Stevens, S.J., Baker, V.H. and Cole, A.T. (1993) Mothers' awareness of HIV and AIDS. *Health Visitor*, 66(12): 443–444.

Tattam, A. (1993) Sex education cuts threaten health aim. *Nursing Times*, 89(1): 8.

Taylor, J. (1994) The sick and well adolescent. In: *Health Promotion and Patient Education*. (Ed. P. Webb) Chapman and Hall, London.

United Kingdom Central Council (1992) *Code of Professional Conduct*. UKCC, London.

Wells, R. (1988) AIDS – are nurses ready to meet the challenge? *Senior Nurse*, 8(1): 6–7.

Woodcock, A., Stenner, K. and Ingham, R. (1992) 'All these contraceptives, videos and that …': Young people talking about sex education. *Health Education Research*, 7(4): 517–315.

Further reading

Henggeler, S., Melton, G. and Rodrigue, J.R. (1992) *Pediatric and Adolescent AIDS*. Sage Publications, Newbury Park.
This book is a useful source of information on HIV and AIDS in children and adolescents. It reviews many studies undertaken in the USA which have relevance for nurses in the UK, particularly those working in the field of health promotion.

Chapter 9
Substance Abuse

Adolescence is a period of life during which individuals make choices about a number of important issues which may have both short and long term consequences upon health. It is also a time when problem solving strategies are developed (Adams and Adams 1991), some of which may be considered to be adaptive and others maladaptive. The misuse of alcohol, tobacco and drugs may be considered to be a maladaptive way of coping with this often stressful stage of the lifespan. However, the use and misuse of such substances is complicated by both political and social norms as well as expectations. Taking a global perspective shows that there are wide variations in views about the use of various substances. Governments throughout the world continue to accumulate revenue from substances which are known to have harmful, if not lethal, effects upon health. The use and abuse of substances must therefore be viewed within both a social and a political context.

The complexity of influences upon adolescents in relation to substance abuse can raise important questions, and present a degree of conflict, for nurses. For example, most nurses are aware of the continuation of media advertising for tobacco and alcohol, and governmental reticence in banning such advertising. The discrepancy between the income earned through the sale of substances such as tobacco and alcohol, and the amount spent on the prevention and treatment of tobacco and alcohol-related disease is vast. Many nurses and other health care professionals find this political stance to be inexplicable.

This chapter will explore some of the issues surrounding the use and abuse of alcohol, tobacco, drugs and solvents during adolescence. The reasons why some adolescents engage in maladaptive behaviour, and the consequences of that behaviour, will be discussed – particularly in relation to preventative health strategies.

The use and abuse of substances

Alcohol

The extent to which adolescents use alcohol, drugs, solvents and tobacco is widely discussed in the literature but does present certain methodological problems for researchers. The prevalence of alcohol use and misuse among adolescents is largely unknown, and research into alcohol use and misuse is fraught with problems. First of all, alcohol consumption is not illegal (although the sale of alcohol has certain restrictions), and alcohol is widely used and socially acceptable. Johnston *et al.* (1989) in a survey in the USA found that the vast majority of young people had tried alcohol by the latter stages of adolescence. Secondly, research into alcohol use among adolescents has usually relied upon self-reporting measures (e.g. Hawker 1978; OPCS 1991), which may be unreliable given that the sale of alcohol to people under the age of 18 is illegal in England, and most States in the USA prohibit the sale of alcohol to people under the age of 21. Research which asks adolescents about the extent to which they will break the law must be viewed with some scepticism. Steinberg (1987) suggests that most people of any age are likely to play down their true alcohol consumption. A third problem exists because alcohol misusers may not present with major health problems, and they may go largely undetected for a number of years. The effects of alcohol upon health are cumulative. Some persistent misusers will eventually find themselves in trouble because of drink driving and antisocial behaviour, but these individuals represent the extreme. Therefore, data about alcohol misuse gathered through the health services or through legal statistics will only represent a small proportion of the overall problem.

The problem then is difficult to define, and we are left to rely on a paucity of data, and a degree of speculation. We have already mentioned that research which relies on self-reporting may be unreliable. In addition, Farrell and Strang (1991), in their review of instruments designed to highlight alcohol related problems, suggest that many existing screening instruments designed for use with adult groups are unsuitable for adolescents, and recently designed instruments for adolescents such as the *Adolescent Alcohol Involvement Scale* and the *Youth Diagnostic Screening Test* require further testing to ensure reliability and internal validity. It is however probably true to say that whilst most young people will try alcohol, the majority treat it with caution and do not habitually misuse it. An OPCS survey (1991) found that 40% of 11–15 year olds in England, had never had a drink, and approximately 30% said that they had a drink a few times per year. 18% said they did so once or twice a month and 13% said they usually drank once or twice a week. It is unfortunately evident that, for a minority of young people, alcohol use becomes a serious and potentially lethal problem. According to Farrell and Strang (1991) the number of young people in this group is increasing.

Drugs

A great deal more is known about the prevalence of illicit drug use, possibly because young people are more likely to come into contact with either the health services or the law, or because for some unknown reason they are more willing to admit to taking drugs than they are to consuming alcohol. A further reason for the advanced state of knowledge may be because the short term consequences of drug use have encouraged more research and have attracted greater funding. The reasons are certainly not clear.

A recent survey of drug misuse in Britain (ISDD 1993) which has drawn on data from both national and regional research, has provided a useful summary of changes in drug use and prevalence. Cannabis is the most commonly tried drug, with prevalence estimated at 1–2% in 12–13 year olds, rising to 15% in 13–16 year olds (Coggans *et al.* 1991; Balding 1992).

Hallucinogens, such as 'magic mushrooms' and LSD are less widely tried than cannabis, but Coggans *et al* (1991) found that, among a group of 13–16 year olds in Scotland, 7% had tried magic mushrooms and 6% had tried LSD. These findings are consistent with those of Balding (1992) who also found that 6–7% of 15–16 year olds had experienced magic mushrooms or LSD. Balding also noted a marked positive correlation with age, and gender differences with more boys admitting experience of these drugs than girls.

This gender difference is reversed in Balding's data relating to amphetamine use, with more girls admitting use than boys. Balding found that just over 5% of his sample had tried amphetamines, a prevalence which was confirmed by Coggans *et al.* (1991) who found, in their subjects from a wider age range, a prevalence of 4%.

The use of cocaine and heroin among school-age adolescents is less than with the hallucinogens and cannabis. Farrell and Strang (1991), in their review of literature from the USA and the UK, show an overall fall in use of these drugs. These findings could be indicative of the availability of less expensive drugs, such as ecstasy, or of increased fear of injecting drugs because of the media focus upon HIV and AIDS. There is however no room for complacency, as around 1% of adolescents in the surveys carried out by Coggans *et al.* (1991) and Balding (1992) admitted trying

cocaine or heroin, and the Gallup/Wrangler survey (cited in ISDD 1993) of
15–24 year olds show an increase of heroin and cocaine use with age.

Whilst cocaine and heroin use among adolescents is apparently falling, there has, as mentioned above, been an increase in the use of
ecstasy over the past five years (ISDD 1993). Available data present a
disturbing picture for those involved in drug prevention. The Scottish
survey undertaken in 1988 (Coggans *et al.* 1991) recorded that 1% of
13–16 year olds had tried ecstasy but, by 1991, 4% of 15–16 year olds had
tried the drug (Balding 1992). An even more disturbing set of data were
generated from a survey in one Liverpool school (cited in ISDD 1993)
which found that 10% of 15–16 year olds had tried ecstasy. Whilst the
Scottish survey involved a sample with a wider age range which therefore limits direct comparison, and the external validity of the Liverpool
study is low, there is clearly a need to monitor ecstasy use very carefully.

The epidemiological data relating to drug use are clearly disturbing,
even more so because of the nature of the research undertaken and the
possibility of under reporting. We have referred to the problems of using
self-report instruments when discussing alcohol use, and similar problems exist in relation to drug use. Farrell and Strang (1991) suggest that
self-report measures should be backed up with physiological measures,
and that instruments designed for use with an adult population should be
adapted and tested for use with younger samples. There are, however, an
increasing number of instruments available for use with adolescent
subjects which have been shown to be reliable (see Farrell and Strang
for a review).

Solvents

Abuse of solvents during early adolescence is a relatively recent phenomenon in Britain, and according to Mangan (1988), emerged as a
problem when the punk rock era highlighted to the media the popular
obsession with self-destruction. The list of relatively common, and legally obtainable, substances that are abused is vast and includes substances such as lighter fuel, glue, aerosols, butane, perfumes, acetone,
dry cleaning fluid and the vapour of burning plastic. The dangers of
abuse are great, particularly during the immediate period of inhalation
and the following period of intoxication. It does not take great imagi-
nation to conclude that placing a plastic bag over the face and inhaling a
substance which makes you feel dizzy and intoxicated carries certain
risks. In addition, there are potential long term effects of solvent abuse
such as damage to the brain, liver and kidneys (ISDD 1988).

Abuse of solvents is more commonly thought of as a group activity
(Strang and Connell 1985) where peer group pressure plays a significant

part. However, some children and adolescents will abuse solvents alone, and according to Gay (1986) these young people are more worrying than those who do so in groups because they use solvents as 'a retreat from adolescence, from family or from life' (p21). Clearly, preventative strategies must take cognisance of these two discrete groups of solvent abusers.

The number of adolescents who have experimented with solvents is probably higher than those who have used cannabis, with surveys showing prevalence of 12% among 13–16 year olds (Coggans *et al.* 1991) in Scotland, and 8% among 15–16 year olds in the Exeter survey (Balding 1992). These variations in prevalence are probably indicative of the use of solvents among younger adolescents, who were included in the sample of the Scottish study. From these data it could be postulated that by 15–16 years of age, adolescents have either moved onto to abuse of a different range of substances, or that they are no longer substance abusing at all. Equally, it could be surmised that there are geographic variations in solvent abuse. Certainly the prevalence of solvent abuse appears to be higher in deprived areas and among children and adolescents who are known to have emotional and behavioural problems (O'Connor 1983; Black 1984).

Smoking

Patterns of cigarette smoking among adolescents have declined since reaching a peak in the 1970s (Conger 1991). Given the known detrimental effects of smoking upon health, however, the estimated 10% of adolescents who continue to smoke regularly (OPCS 1991) represent a significant challenge to health educators.

Trends in smoking have also highlighted interesting and inexplicable gender differentials, both in terms of the age at which smoking starts and in the decrease in smoking patterns. Boys are more likely to start smoking at a younger age than girls, although by the age of 13 years, girls effectively 'catch up' (Stewart and Orme 1989; OPCS 1991). The reason for this difference is interesting, but may only be a reflection of greater independence afforded to boys by parents, giving them more opportunity to experiment. Additionally, the overall decline in cigarette smoking has been more marked among adolescent boys than among girls. The result has been a greater prevalence in smoking among girls (Conger 1991), although it is interesting that more boys actually experiment with cigarettes and then give up (Goddard 1989).

Gender differences in the prevalence of smoking are difficult to explain and clearly further research is needed into this important area. Several explanations have been suggested however. Stewart and Orme

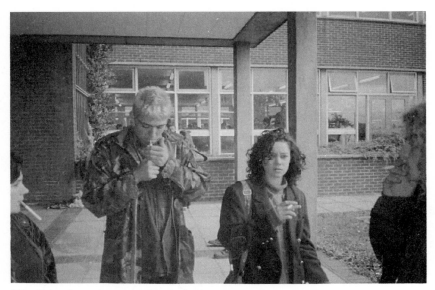

Fig. 9.1   An estimated 10% of adolescents smoke regularly.

(1991) propose that boys give up smoking because of concern with 'limitations smoking may place on athletic prowess', whilst girls smoke 'to try and regulate their weight or to emulate a "cool", sexually attractive woman' (p154). Conger (1991) proposes an alternative view and suggests that adolescent girls do not perceive themselves to be as vulnerable as their male counterparts, because historically smoking-related diseases have been more prevalent among men. Conger (1991) also places some blame for smoking among adolescent girls at the door of the media, who he suggests target younger women. Whatever the reasons for the gender differences in smoking behaviour, it does appear that adolescent boys and girls may smoke for different reasons and may be influenced by different factors. These differences may be important in terms of preventative strategies, and, as suggested above, further research is warranted.

Factors which influence the use and abuse of substances

There are a number of factors which appear to influence the use of substances during adolescence, several of which are inextricably related. This section will look at the influence of parents, peers, personality, the social environment and finally the possibility of genetic influences.

Parental influence

The role of social learning in terms of adolescent behaviour has been discussed in Chapter 5. According to Bandura (1977), children and adolescents learn many of their behaviours, as well as their internal value systems, from their observations of others, and by monitoring the consequences of overt behaviours which Bandura referred to as 'vicarious learning'. Parents are clearly influential in this process and their behaviours and beliefs are thought to be significant in terms of substance abuse.

Hawker (1978), in a large study of 7306 adolescents in England between the ages of 13–18 years, provided valuable data relating to adolescent drinking. While this study is now dated, it continues to have importance because of the very large and representative sample used. One of the most influential factors upon adolescent drinking found in Hawker's study related to parental drinking behaviour. Adolescent drinkers were more likely to have parents who drink alcohol, a finding which is supported by more recent research (Conger 1991; Farrell and Strang 1991).

Drug taking among adolescents appears to be similarly influenced by parental behaviour. Advances in pharmaceutics mean that there are pills for virtually all ailments, and children frequently observe adults taking medication when they are unwell. Indeed most children will at some time take medication themselves when they are ill, and are reinforced in their behaviour by feeling better. Medication is clearly not only available for physical complaints, but also for psychological dysfunction, including minor depression, anxiety and insomnia. If adolescents observe parents taking medication (albeit legally) in order to help them cope with the stresses of life, it is perhaps not surprising that they may attempt to cope with their own stress by taking drugs, particularly if they do not possess alternative coping skills. Oppenheimer (1985) suggests that drug taking by parents and other close adults can serve as a role model for adolescents. This may be an over simplistic view, and clearly not all adolescents whose parents take medication will abuse drugs themselves. However, there is some evidence which suggests that parental use of barbiturates, amphetamines and tranquillizers, in particular, is correlated with illegal drug use during adolescence (Conger 1991). The use of alcohol as a coping mechanism by parents is also correlated with drug use (Farrell and Strang 1991; Beardslee, *et al.* 1986).

The way in which children and adolescents model themselves on their parents also applies to smoking, with the children of smoking parents being twice as likely to smoke as children whose parents do not smoke (Conger 1991; Stewart and Orme 1991). An OPCS survey (1991) found that siblings too appear to provide role models and sibling smokers were found to be even more influential than parents. Adolescents who had at least one brother or sister who smoked were 4–5 times more likely to be smokers themselves than those who did not. An interesting paper by Doherty and Whitehead (1986), which investigated the social dynamics of smoking within a family context, observed that smoking can signal a number of behaviours, such as talking, relaxing, seeking solitude, stating independence, showing distress and belonging. It could be postulated that children learn that the cue for these important functions is a cigarette. Thus for some children and adolescents cigarettes are seen to play a powerful role in family dynamics.

Just as parental behaviour in relation to alcohol, drugs and smoking can provide a detrimental role model for children and adolescents, so too can parental attitudes serve as a positive role model. Hawker (1978), in her early research on adolescent drinking, identified that parental approval of alcohol could influence the frequency of adolescent drinking. Those adolescents in the sample who had first been introduced to alcohol at home were less likely to drink frequently than those who had experienced their first drink in a public house. For those introduced to alcohol at home, alcohol did not become a 'forbidden fruit'. Hawker suggested that:

'if drinking commences at an early age in circumstances where deception is necessary, it can be seen that for some, drinking is associated from the onset with deviant behaviour' (p22).

Parental approval of alcohol, and allowing alcohol to be consumed in moderation *openly* may then reduce the frequency of consumption. Furthermore, Hawker concludes that parents are possibly the best people to introduce alcohol to adolescents, particularly if parents have a responsible attitude towards alcohol themselves.

Parental views can also influence drug taking among adolescents. Adolescents whose parents strongly and overtly disapprove of drug taking are less likely to engage in drug use (see Conger 1991), and those who have a relationship with parents which involves democracy and trust are less likely to become habitual users (Newcomb and Bentler 1988).

Peer influence

A second major influence upon substance use during adolescence relates to peer influence, which has been implicated in relation to abuse of alcohol, drugs, solvents and smoking.

In relation to alcohol, a study by Smith and Collins (1989) found that 93% of 16–18 year olds had started drinking as a result of peer pressure. The earlier study by Hawker (1978) had also found a correlation between adolescent drinking and peer affiliation. Belonging to one or more social or leisure organizations was likely to increase the frequency of drinking, although it is likely that these data represent greater opportunity for drinking, and the need for adolescents to form independent relationships and find a social identity. Public houses have for many years been places where young people can meet, talk freely and socialize away from parents and siblings. Indeed in some areas, a lack of facilities for young people, mean that public houses are the *only* places young people can meet away from the home.

Using substances as a means of gaining entry to a peer group has been cited in relation to smoking (Nash 1987; Tones *et al.* 1990), and drugs (Pallikkathayil and Tweed 1983). Adolescents appear to have a need to belong, and peer groups have an important function in enabling adolescents to gain independence (see Chapter 2). For some adolescents making friends and associating with a peer group is difficult and some adolescents may find that the only way to 'belong' is to conform to the behaviours and practices of a particular group. There is however some debate here, and it is difficult to ascertain whether adolescents abuse a substance in order to join a group, or whether their wish to engage in solvent abuse leads them to seek out peers with similar wishes. As we have discussed earlier in this book, the need for peer group affiliation appears to diminish with age. It is interesting to note, however, that in relation to drug taking the peer group remains important throughout the drug taker's life (Oppenheimer 1985), possibly because drug takers will always require a network of people in order to ensure their supply of drugs.

Societal views and the media

A third influence on substance abuse during adolescence relates to societal views and media promotion of various substances, whether overtly through advertising, or covertly through fiction. We have already referred to the current practice of taking 'pills for all ills', and certainly society must take some of the blame for promoting the view that medication is available for a whole host of problems including being unable to cope with stress. A further problem relates to the view that certain activities such as smoking and drinking are 'adult'.

In the United Kingdom, Parry-Jones (1985) suggests that smoking and drinking have become 'universal symbols of maturity' (p588). The tradition of using alcohol to mark special occasions such as adult birthdays, weddings and other celebrations reinforces this view. The use of alcohol is also frequently portrayed within the media as being both desirable and sociable, and public houses are portrayed, particularly on the television, as being places to meet friends and socialize. Popular British 'soap operas' portray the public house as being the normal place to go at lunch time and after work. Whilst we assume that this portrayal is designed to facilitate the story line, it does perhaps give a somewhat distorted view of the importance of public houses in the community. A further use of alcohol frequently demonstrated by the media and by adults is as a coping mechanism. It is not unusual for adults to offer each other a drink if they are feeling depressed, emotional or shocked which may represent to the adolescent an acceptable way of coping with stress and distress.

Personality

A further potential influence upon substance use is the personality of the adolescent, although data remain conflicting and considerable differences of opinion persist (Farrell and Strang 1991). Clearly there are several groups of adolescents to consider in any discussion of substance abuse. There are those who never experiment with alcohol, drugs, solvents or tobacco; those who experiment but who do not become persistent or problem users; and a minority, but still significant number of adolescents, for whom substances become a way of life. Personality-related factors reflecting maladjustment have been postulated as an explanation for these differences.

The concept of a particular personality type being prone to substance abuse is interesting and controversial. Khantzian (1985) proposed that some individuals have what can be described as a 'disturbed personality' making them more prone to using drugs to cope with difficulties. Gross (1992) discusses the possibility of a 'conforming' personality which may be important in relation to the efficacy of peer influence. Clearly, depending upon the peer group, conformity can be either positive or negative. Oppenheimer (1985) also discusses certain personality traits which are characteristic of drug users. These include high rebelliousness and low obedience. Rebelliousness was also found to be a factor in predicting cigarette smoking (Conger 1991). Parry-Jones (1985) suggests that adolescents who become dependent are likely to be immature, and have a low self-concept. Studies which have looked at extroversion and introversion as predictors of substance abuse have provided data which are less conclusive. Oppenheimer (1985), in a review of research into the personality characteristics of drug takers, found that findings were conflicting. Depression has been found to be correlated with substance abuse, but problems exist in relation to defining causal relationships, particularly in relation to alcohol and drug abuse. Whether adolescents use substances because they are depressed, or whether excessive use of alcohol or drugs leads to depression, is unclear. However, a relationship does appear to exist, and the more depressed the adolescent the more likely they are to become intoxicated and choose negative coping strategies (Adams and Adams 1991).

Genetic links

One final influence which is worthy of consideration here relates to the genetic basis for problem drinking. We have already referred to parental influence on drinking behaviour, but have considered that influence only in relation to parental approval minimizing deviance and to adolescents modelling parental drinking patterns. The possibility of substance dependence being innate is both interesting and complex, as well as being somewhat controversial, possibly because there exists a paucity of data to date. Several research approaches have been attempted involving twin studies, adoption studies, and gene probes, particularly in relation to alcohol dependence (see Rutter *et al.* 1990). Because of the small samples involved, such studies are inconclusive; but future work may well throw further light on the genetic link.

In conclusion, we can say that there appear to be a number of factors which influence adolescent substance use, although what is not clear is why some adolescents develop dependence on substances whereas others may experiment and give up, or in the case of alcohol be able to drink in moderation. Personality and genetic factors may play a part, and parental attitude and peer influence appear to be significant. What is clearly needed, however, is further research into the relationship between these potentially influencing variables.

The role of the nurse in substance abuse

So far in this chapter we have looked at the prevalence of substance abuse and at various factors which are influential in the use and abuse of substances by adolescents. Clearly one of the most effective ways of minimizing the detrimental effects of substance abuse is to discourage young people from ever experimenting with substances at all or, in the case of alcohol, to encourage a sensible attitude towards use. Failing that, it is important that those who are closely involved with adolescents, including parents and health professionals, should possess skills which enable them to identify early signs of abuse, and be aware of how to mobilize appropriate intervention.

Preventative and interventive strategies are in reality extremely complex however, for a number of reasons. Firstly, preventive education is always taking place within a social climate which projects to the adolescent a variety of inconsistencies relating to substance use and abuse. Secondly, there is little empirical evidence which can inform the most effective ways of prevention or intervention in relation to substance abuse. Whilst preventative strategies can be and have been evaluated in the short term, longitudinal research is needed in order to ascertain the most effective ways of ensuring long term positive behaviour. Thirdly, the changing face of the school system in the United Kingdom, and the roles of health professionals within that system, makes it difficult to undertake research which has adequate internal and external validity. Since most preventative activity takes place within the school system, these changes have important implications for future research. Finally, in terms of effective interventions, there remains a paucity of research into the efficacy of the treatment of substance abuse among adolescents. This lack of research is partially reflective of the lack of facilities nationally, which are aimed specifically at the treatment of young abusers (Farrell and Strang 1991). We are left then with a limited amount of specific research into the best ways of preventing and treating substance abuse among adolescents. Clearly, this situation is undesirable, both in terms of helping nurses who are involved in the prevention of substance abuse among adolescents and in terms of the brevity of the current state of substance abuse among adolescents. There is however a substantial amount of literature which looks at health promotion in relation to substance abuse, and it is to that literature that we now turn.

Farrell and Strang (1991), in their review of substance abuse among adolescents, discuss the age at which preventative strategies should be started. We have seen in the discussion of the prevalence of substance abuse in the early part of this chapter that, by the start of adolescence, smoking (particularly among boys) and solvent abuse are not uncommon. The age at which initiation into drug use occurs is also declining. Farrell and Strang suggest that preventative strategies should therefore be considered among primary school children. Clearly school nurses and teachers are the ideal people to undertake such a role, although we recognize that teachers already have a full curriculum and additional demands on their time may lead to some conflict. Care should also be taken to ensure that education is sensitive in terms of age and cognitive development (see Chapter 5). The view of encouraging prevention in primary schools is reiterated in relation to smoking prevention by Stewart and Orme (1989).

The social context within which health promotion takes place is also discussed in the literature in relation to preventing substance abuse. We have already discussed a number of factors which influence substance abuse among adolescents and it is important that preventive strategies are geared towards these factors (Stewart and Orme 1989). The Advisory Council on the Misuse of Drugs (1993) discusses the importance of health promotion in schools which is sensitive to these factors, which has relevance to all forms of substance abuse. They propose that the following considerations should be taken into account.

1. *The audience* The efficacy of health promotion will be influenced by age, characteristics, experience and the social background of the adolescent.
2. *The environment* The efficacy of health promotion will vary according to the community in which the school is situated e.g. the availability of drugs within the community.
3. *The prevention strategy* Programmes of prevention which are aimed at the community as well as at individuals will have higher efficacy. A preventative programme should therefore account for wider factors which influence abuse.
4. *Level of provision* The amount of training given to the teachers (and school nurses), the amount of time given to preventative activities, the quality of the delivery and the amount of resources allocated to the preventative programme will clearly influence its efficacy.
5. *Delivery of education* It is important that educational processes for the delivery of preventative strategies correspond with those activities which were actually planned. The Advisory Council recommend that more attention should be given to the evaluation of *processes* as well as outcomes.
6. *Behavioural outcomes* Programmes aimed at the prevention of use, delay in use, safety in use, decreasing the quantity and frequency of use of specific drugs may be more effective than programmes which are generalistic in nature.

In line with this philosophy, and in recognition of the changing role of the school nurse, partially brought about by the NHS and Community Care Act (1990), Holt (1990) discusses the need for school nurses to adapt their work to take account of the individual student and the social context within which they function. Holt describes a system of assessment which has five objectives which include the provision of a health profile for each child, and a health profile of the school. The consideration of the individual student within the school context is vital if health promotion is to be effective. We have already discussed demographic variations in substance abuse and preventative strategies must account for the different circumstances within which adolescents function. This point is emphasized by Levin (1989) who stresses that:

> 'Strategies ... must take account of factors in the wider social and political context which affect young people's struggle to survive, grow, be caring and be cared about' (p152).

This is not to say, however, that any school (or indeed school nurse or parent) should feel complacent because the community is not renowned for substance abuse. Situations can change rapidly, and certainly in relation to smoking and alcohol use and abuse demography appears to play little part. It is important that the school milieu and the community are supportive of health promotion strategies that are taking place within a school. Continuing to encourage schools to adopt a 'no smoking' policy among staff, for example, may well assist in ensuring that teachers become positive role models rather than negative ones, and reiterating information to shopkeepers about the sale of solvents, tobacco and alcohol can reinforce the message being put forward by the school to adolescents who try to purchase such substances.

The focus of health promotion is also clearly important in preventing substance abuse among adolescents. The Advisory Council on the Abuse of Drugs (1993) suggests that strategies which are sustained and intensive and which teach decision-making and life skills are more likely to be effective than didactic approaches. This point is also emphasized by Tones *et al.* (1990) who suggest that health promotion activity should be geared towards effective decision making, self-empowerment and promoting basic coping skills. Part of this approach is encouraging adolescents to be discerning about the information they receive from variety of sources:

> 'Pupils should know how to distinguish between fact, promotion and polemic, and how to weigh and interpret information about health ...' (p97).

Although there is little research about the efficacy of preventative strategies there is even less about how to intervene with adolescents who are suspected of, or who are known to be, abusing substances.

The implication for nurses

Clearly those nurses involved with adolescents must be aware of warning signs which are indicative of substance abuse. Such signs may include sores around the mouth and nose in the case of solvent abuse, lack of interest in school work, loss of concentration etc. Developing a trusting relationship with the adolescent can enable sensitive and non-confrontational questioning about what is wrong. It is also important that parents are aware of these signs and even more important that they know where they can go for help and advice if they suspect that something is wrong. This first point of contact may be with the school nurse. Thus local knowledge about where to refer parents is vital. Apart from the school, parents may contact the GP or practice nurse, particularly if health promotion material is freely available in health centres and surgeries. Being able to follow up the advice given in promotional material is extremely important, and we would urge nurses working in general practice to be absolutely cognisant of the services they offer, either directly or indirectly.

Research relating to intervention in cases of known substance abuse is, as we have already mentioned, scarce. There remain few treatment centres specifically designed for adolescents and Farrell and Strang (1991) warn of the effects of incorporating adolescents into programmes designed for adults. What most authors are in agreement on is that in view of the importance of the social context in adolescent substance abuse it is important that intervention is aimed towards not only the individual but also the family and other significant people in the lives of affected adolescents (Watson 1986; Steinberg 1987). Most intervention relies upon behavioural modification, the development of social skills, diversionary activities, remedial teaching and psychotherapy (Watson 1986; see Strang and Connell 1985) within a context of family therapy.

References

Adams, M. and Adams, J. (1991) Life events, depression and perceived problem solving alternatives in adolescents. *Journal of Child Psychology and Psychiatry*, 32(5): 811–820

Advisory Council on the Misuse of Drugs (1993) *Drug Education in Schools: The Need for New Impetus*. HMSO, London.

Balding, J. (1992) *Young People in 1991*. Schools Health Education Unit, University of Exeter.

Bandura, A. (1977) *Social Learning Theory*. Prentice Hall, New Jersey.

Beardslee, W.R., Son, L. and Vaillant, G.E. (1986) Exposure to parental alcoholism during childhood and outcome in adulthood: a prospective longitudinal study. *British Journal of Psychiatry*, 149: 584–591.

Black, D. (1984) Glue sniffing – the facts. *Midwife, Health Visitor and Community Nurse*, 20: 21–22.

Coggans, N. *et al.* (1991) *National Evaluation of Drug Education in Scotland.* ISDD

Conger, J.J. (1991) *Adolescence and Youth*, 4th edn. Harper Collins, New York.

Doherty, W.J. and Whitehead, D.A. (1986) The social dynamics of cigarette smoking: A family systems perspective. *Family Process Inc*, 25: 453–459.

Farrell, M. and Strang, J. (1991) Substance use and misuse in childhood and adolescence. *Journal of Child Psychology and Psychiatry*, 32(1): 109–128.

Gay, M. (1986) Drug and solvent use in adolescents. *Nursing Times*, 82: 21–22.

Goddard, E. (1989) *Smoking among Adolescent School Children in England 1988.* HMSO, London.

Gross, R.D. (1992) *Psychology: The Science of Mind and Behaviour*, 2nd edn. Hodder and Stoughton, London.

Hawker, A. (1978) *Adolescents and Alcohol.* Edsall, London.

Holt, H. (1990) Southampton Health Appraisal pilot study. *Nursing Standard*, 4(16): 26–31.

ISDD (1988) *Drug Misuse – A Basic Briefing.* HMSO, London.

ISDD (1993) *National Audit of Drug Misuse in Britain.* College Hill Press, London.

Johnston, L.D., O'Malley, P.M. and Bachman, J.G. (1989) *Drug Use, Drinking and Smoking: National Survey Results from High School, College and Young Adult Populations 1975–1988.* NIDA, Washington DC.

Khantzian, E.J. (1985) The self medication hypothesis of addictive disorders: focus on heroin and cocaine dependence. *American Journal of Psychiatry*, 142: 1259–1264.

Levin, L.S. (1989) Health for today's youth, hope for tomorrow's world. *World Health Forum*, 10: 1551–1557.

Mangan, P. (1988) Solvent abuse. *Nursing Standard*, 2(46): 28–29.

Nash, J. (1987) Sparking up – smoking and style in school. *Health Education Journal*, 46: 152–155.

Newcomb, M.D. and Bentler, P.M. (1988) *Consequences of Adolescent Drug Use: Impact on the Lives of Young Adults.* Sage, Newbury Park, California.

O'Connor, D. (1983) *Glue Sniffing and Volatile Substances: Case Studies of Children and Young Adults.* Gower, Aldershot.

OPCS (1991) *Smoking among Secondary School Children in 1990.* HMSO, London.

Oppenheimer, E. (1985) Drug taking. In: *Child and Adolescent Psychiatry: Modern Approaches*, 2nd edn. (Eds M. Rutter and L. Hersov). Blackwell Scientific Publications, Oxford.

Pallikkathayil, L. and Tweed, S. (1983) Substance abuse: alcohol and drugs during adolescence. *Nursing Clinics of North America*, 18(2): 313–321.

Parry-Jones, W.L. (1985) Adolescent disturbance. In: *Child and Adolescent Psychiatry: Modern Approaches*, 2nd edn. (Eds M. Rutter and L. Hersov). Blackwell Scientific Publications, Oxford.

Rutter, M., MacDonald, H., LeCouteur, A., Harrington, R., Bolton, P. and Bailey, A. (1990) Genetic factors in child psychiatric disorders II. *Journal of Child Psychology and Psychiatry*, 31: 39–83.

Smith, I. and Collins, F. (1989) Patterns of Drug Abuse. *Nursing Times*, 85(10): 55.

Steinberg, D. (1987) *Basic Adolescent Psychiatry*. Blackwell Scientific Publications, Oxford.

Stewart, A.J. and Orme, J. (1989) Teenage smoking and health. *Health Visitor*, 62(3): 91–94.

Stewart, A.J. and Orme, J. (1991) Why do adolescents smoke? In: *Child Care: Some Nursing Perspectives*. (Ed. A. Glasper) Wolfe, London.

Strang, J. and Connell, P. (1985) Clinical aspects of drug and alcohol abuse. In: *Child and Adolescent Psychiatry: Modern Approaches*, 2nd edn. (Eds M. Rutter and L. Hersov) Blackwell Scientific Publications, Oxford.

Tones, K., Tilford, S. and Robinson, Y. (1990) *Health Education: Effectiveness and Efficiency*. Chapman and Hall, London.

Watson, J.M. (1986) *Solvent Abuse*. Croom Helm, London.

Further reading

Tones, K., Tilford, S. and Robinson, Y. (1990) *Health Education: Effectiveness and Efficiency*. Chapman and Hall, London.
This excellent health education book gives practical detail about working with adolescents in school and smoking prevention.

Chapter 10
Suicide and Parasuicide During Adolescence

Death during childhood and adolescence is always seen as tragic, but never more so than when the death occurs due to deliberate self-harm on the part of the young person. Fortunately, such occurrences are relatively rare, although suicide does comprise a significant number of deaths, particularly during late adolescence (OPCS 1992). There is also evidence to suggest that suicide rates among adolescents are rising (DoH 1992). Perhaps, the most difficult aspect of suicide deaths is that they should be entirely preventable, and consequently the guilt felt by parents, friends and involved professionals is immense. These feelings are also apparent when adolescents attempt suicide.

This chapter aims to explore adolescent suicide and parasuicide, in an attempt to enable nurses involved with adolescents to understand why some adolescents engage in suicide behaviour. This exploration inevitably involves discussion of psychological theory relating to the evolving identity of the adolescent, and discussion of depression and its role in suicide behaviour. The chapter also includes data relating to the identification of potentially 'at risk' adolescents, exploration of approaches aimed at preventing adolescent suicide, and aspects of caring for parasuicidal adolescents.

The search for identity

We have already referred to the work of Erikson (1965) and the later expansion of Erikson's theories by Marcia (1982) in Chapter 4. Marcia suggests that adolescents establish identity through processes of crisis and commitment. Crises are periods when the adolescent is faced with resolving issues relating to personal goals and values, whereas commitment refers to the decision-making processes which lead the adolescent towards a specific goal or belief, after consideration of alternatives. A crisis will therefore be resolved by making a commitment.

Marcia argued that each adolescent will be faced with varying crises and commitments, but that some adolescents will never experience crises, and some will experience crises but will be unable to resolve them.

If adolescents are searching for personal identity, then they do so within complex social situations which influence crisis resolution. The social world of the adolescent usually includes parents, peers, school, and may include other influences such as religious affiliation and membership of other social groups. Grotevant and Cooper (1985) suggest that the role of the parents is important in terms of personal identity. Adolescents who are able to communicate well with their parents, and who do not experience criticism of their views are more likely to develop a clear sense of personal identity. Peers are also strongly influential, particularly during early and middle adolescence, and the adolescent may develop strong and often intense relationships with one or more of their peers. These friendships act as important buffers particularly during crisis periods and Youniss and Smollar (1985) found in their study that adolescents are more likely to share their worries, views and conflicts with a close friend, than with any one else. Friendships do however tend to vary in their intensity, function and quality throughout the process of adolescence (see Chapter 4).

Suicide behaviour

Knowledge of the adolescent's crises in the search for identity and the influence of the social world of the adolescent gives us a basis for hypothesizing about suicide behaviour. Most adolescents in their search for identity will move in and out of crisis periods which require resolution. That is not to say that all adolescents who fail to resolve crises will engage in suicide behaviour, neither are we suggesting that the crises are the cause of suicide behaviour. What we are suggesting is that periods of crisis for which the adolescent cannot find resolution can leave *some* adolescents with a sense of emptiness and depression. These feelings may accumulate over a relatively long period of time, with the adolescent attempting unsuccessfully to solve problems and achieve a sense of identity (Seligman and Peterson 1986). The sense of self brought along from childhood is lost and there is nothing to replace lost values and beliefs. Conger (1991) likens the ensuing depression to a state of mourning and suggests that most adolescent suicide attempts are the result 'of a long series of unsuccessful attempts to find solutions to difficulties' (p556).

The scope of the problem

The incidence of suicide is rare in childhood and adolescence but it has been recognized for some time that it is on the increase (Hempel 1992), and rises with age. Over the past ten years in England and Wales rates for male adolescent suicide have steadily risen (OPCS 1983–1993). The rates for females have remained relatively stable. In England and Wales, the ratio of male adolescent suicides to females suicides in approximately 4:1 in the 15–19 age range. Tables 10.1 and 10.2 show the number of deaths and the rate of deaths per million for suicides in England and Wales.

There are also cultural and geographic differences in suicide, which were first recognized in a famous study by Durkheim (1952), who showed that suicide rates varied between social groups. Later statistics by the World Health Organization (1990) showed that suicide is a more frequent cause of death in some countries than in others. Religious, ethnic and economic variables also appear to be significant. In the USA white males are more likely to succeed in suicide, and white females are more likely to make unsuccessful attempts (Conger 1991).

The extent of attempted suicide is unknown as not all parasuicides are referred for treatment and some adolescents do not even report their attempts to their parents (Walker *et al.* 1990). What is clear is that all attempted suicides should be taken seriously (Parry-Jones 1985; Steinberg 1987) as many adolescents who succeed in suicide have a history of previous attempts. An early study by Shaffer (1974), which studied the inquest reports of 30 suicides under the age of 15 years in

Table 10.1 Numbers of adolescent suicides by age and gender for 1987–1992

Year			*10–14 years*	*15–19 years*
1987	M	4		103
	F	2		25
1988	M	3		113
	F	1		28
1989	M	1		94
	F	0		20
1990	M	2		100
	F	0		23
1991	M	2		97
	F	1		28
1992	M	1		87
	F	0		23

Source: OPCS Mortality Statistics 1983–1993.

Table 10.2 Death rates by suicide and self-inflicted injury per million for England and Wales 1985–1992 for the age categories 5–14 and 15–24 years, by gender

Year			*5–14 years*	*15–24 years*
1985	M	1		82
	F	0		18
1986	M	1		87
	F	0		20
1987	M	1		93
	F	1		21
1988	M	1		110
	F	0		25
1989	M	0		103
	F	0		19
1990	M	1		117
	F	0		20
1991	M	1		108
	F	0		22
1992	M	—		115
	F	—		21

Source: OPCS Mortality Statistics 1983–1993.

England and Wales, found that about half of child and adolescent suicides had threatened, talked about or attempted suicide within the 24 hours preceding their death.

There are significant gender differences in adolescent suicide behaviour. Boys are more likely to harm themselves using violent methods such as hanging or using firearms which possibly accounts for the higher success rate, whereas girls tend to choose more passive methods such as overdosage of drugs and poisons (Hempel 1992; OPCS 1992). Boys are also more likely to self-harm using gases, vapours and motor vehicle exhaust gas (OPCS 1989, 1991, 1992). Table 10.3 shows gender differences in suicide behaviour.

The warning signs

Various studies have suggested that a number of life events may be associated with suicide behaviour in adolescents (see Shaffer 1985; Mussen *et al.* 1990; Adams and Adams 1991). These events can best be summarized as follows:

- depression;
- family factors;

Table 10.3 Numbers of suicide by selected method and gender in the 15–19 year old category for 1987, 1989, 1991

Method		1987	1989	1991
Poisoning by solid or liquid substance	M	14	12	9
	F	15	8	14
Poisoning by gases and vapours	M	24	20	20
	F	2	2	3
Motor vehicle exhaust gas	M	*	17	19
	F	*	2	1
Hanging	M	43	31	2
	F	3	7	1
Firearms and explosives	M	6	10	5
	F	0	0	1
Jumping from a high place	M	6	7	4
	F	2	0	3

Source: OPCS 1989, 1991, 1993.

* Data unavailable

- loss of a friend;
- physical/sexual abuse;
- substance abuse;
- school factors.

Depression

We have already referred to the cumulative effects of failure to resolve crises which can, for some adolescents, contribute to the onset of depression, which is the most consistently cited precipitating factor associated with adolescent (and adult) suicide (Hodgman and McAnarney 1992). Estimates of the incidence of depression during adolescence are, however, remarkably high. Reynolds (1989) found depression rates in adolescents ranging from 10% to over 30% in various populations, and Donovan and McCarthy (1988) in a survey of 16 and 17 years olds from a general practice population identified their most usual problems as being obesity, depression and acne. These data suggest that depression is a major cause of morbidity during adolescence and, whilst not all depressed adolescents will engage in suicide behaviour, Lowenstein (1990) and Myers *et al.* (1991) suggest that any form of depressive illness should be considered as a sign of potential suicide. Pfeffer *et al.* (1989) add further weight to this argument in their comparison of four groups of adolescents; suicidal only; suicidal – assaultive; assaultive only; and non-suicidal – non-assaultive. They found that the suicidal only group had a higher incidence of depressive disorder than the other groups.

Recognizing depression in adolescents is not always easy, and is rarely as obvious as depression in adulthood, due in part to the signs being confounded by the general changes that tend to take place during this stage of life. However, sleep disorders, eating disturbances, as well as social withdrawal and isolation are frequent signs of depression in adolescents and should all be taken seriously by parents and health care professionals who become aware of such problems (Mussen *et al.* 1990; Conger 1991).

Family factors

It is clearly difficult to determine the extent to which family factors contribute to the onset of depression during adolescence or on the other hand the extent to which adolescent depression contributes to the breakdown of communication within the family, and further research is needed to clarify the association between these two variables. What is apparent, however, is that family factors appear to have significance in terms of adolescent suicide behaviour.

The study by Pfeffer *et al.* (1989) which compared four groups of adolescents admitted to a large voluntary psychiatric hospital in the United States, found differences between adolescents showing suicide behaviour only, and those who showed assaultive and suicidal behaviour. Those showing suicide only behaviour were more likely to have deficit parent/child interaction whereas those showing suicidal and assaultive behaviour were more likely to have witnessed assaultive behaviour in close relatives.

Mussen *et al.* (1990) discuss the importance of communication within the family and suggest that breakdown between the adolescent and significant others is a factor in suicide and parasuicide and Conger (1991) suggests that conflict between parents and the adolescent is also significant. The suicide of a relative is also cited by Conger (1991) as being associated with suicide behaviour in adolescence, although Pfeffer *et al.* (1989) found no significant differences in their four adolescent groups in relation to parental suicide. The death of a parent or relative was however felt to be significant by Adams and Adams (1991).

Fear of parents finding out about truancy and 'anti-social acts' was found by Shaffer (1974) to be the most frequently cited reason for suicide in an early study of inquest records of 30 suicides under the age of 15 years. Shaffer also found that in over half of his sample there was a family history of referred psychological dysfunctioning. Clearly family dynamics may be important in adolescent suicide, although why family factors will lead some adolescents to end, or attempt to end, their lives because of some breakdown in family functioning is uncertain. In terms of preventing suicide behaviour in adolescents, identifying problems within the family poses difficulties for health care professionals. Many families experience conflict and it is an unlikely reason for parents, or adolescents, to seek help. Society expects that such problems should be dealt with within the confines of family. Perhaps given the rise in suicide behaviour and the substantial amount of accumulated knowledge relating to the problems of adolescence there is a need to actively help families to work through some of the traumas which may contribute to communication difficulties. A model for this was attempted by one secondary school in England which invited parents to health education sessions where they could openly discuss, in an informal environment, aspects of adolescence which were worrying or problematic (Gunn 1987). Encouraging parents, who may be experiencing living with an adolescent for the first time, to discuss openly what life is like for them – and to find out that they are not isolated – is a small, but significant, move in the right direction. It seems somewhat ironic that we teach professionals who are involved with children and adolescents about how to communicate effectively with them, and yet we expect parents to have such knowledge by instinct.

Loss of a friend

Friendship is an important factor during adolescence, and patterns of friendship vary in their intensity as the period of adolescence progresses. In early and middle adolescence friendships tend to be intense and dependent, whereas in late adolescence, for most adolescents the intense nature of friendship decreases and is more independent (Selman 1981). We have already mentioned that friends become an important buffer, who can provide a reference group with whom the adolescent can identify. They also provide reinforcement in terms of behaviour and crisis resolution.

The loss of a friend through argument, through changing schools, moving house, or exceptionally if a friend dies, can result in the removal of the buffer. Adams and Adams (1991) suggest that breaking up with a girlfriend/boyfriend is significant in terms of suicide behaviour, as is moving to a new school and the death of a friend. Conflict with friends was also found to be significant by Pfeffer *et al.* (1989) in adolescents who had attempted suicide and McClure (1988) found an association between rejection by friends and suicide. Conger (1991) also suggests that rejection by a friend, and the breaking up of a romance, are important factors in suicide behaviour.

The intensity of friendship and the number of friends may also be important in terms of suicide behaviour. Curran (1987) in a study of suicide and friendship suggested that adolescents exhibiting suicide behaviour were more likely to have fewer close friends, but the friendships they did have were very intense. Adolescents with no friends also give cause for concern given the importance of friendship during adolescence. Whilst some adolescents appear to have no need for friends, and are able to develop a strong sense of identity without reference to same-age peers, they are in the minority and most adolescents appear to rely on the support of friends. Adolescents who are without this support are more likely to develop psychopathology in adulthood (Hartup 1989), and Laufer (1974), in an early but nevertheless interesting text, suggests that the absence of friends should be taken seriously by parents and professionals. Laufer cites an interview with the parents of one adolescent boy who attempted suicide who had not felt his lack of friends was significant until after his suicide attempt.

'He never had many friends. Sometimes he might come home with another boy, but usually a friend would last a week or so. Most of the time he was his own. We ourselves never knew much about mental troubles so we didn't think there was too much wrong if our boy stayed home' (p51).

Clearly the importance of friendship during adolescence should not be under estimated. The intense friendships of the adolescent are important and the loss of such a friendship can lead the bereft adolescent to extreme behaviour, including suicide. Adolescents with no friends should also be considered to be potentially at risk of psychopathology and efforts made to explore why they have no friends and if the lack of friends is an important issue for them.

Associations with physical and sexual abuse

Several studies have found an association between physical and sexual abuse, and suicidal thoughts and behaviour (Deykin *et al.* 1985; Briere *et al.* 1988; Singer 1989; Watkins and Bentovim, 1992). Research into physical and sexual abuse in children and adolescents, however, is problematic by its very nature. Shame and secrecy surround this taboo subject which can lead to stigmatization of the victim and the family. It is also evident that physical and sexual abuse rarely takes place in isolation from other problems within the family and the environment.

There is however some evidence to suggest that sexual abuse can be predictive of suicidal behaviour. McCormack *et al.* (1986), in their study of runaways, found an increased incidence of suicidal feelings among abused adolescents when compared with non-abused adolescents. Likewise, Singer (1989), in a study of men who had been the victims of incest as children, found that suicidal behaviour was not uncommon. Briere *et al.* (1988) also found that previously abused men and women were more likely to have attempted suicide that non-abused controls. An earlier study by Goodwin (1981) found an interesting association between the abuser and suicide attempt by the abused. In a study of sexual abuse in families, eight female victims attempted suicide, all of whom had been abused by their fathers.

Physical abuse is also associated with suicide behaviour. The study by Pfeffer *et al* (1989), which compared four groups of adolescents including a suicidal group and a suicidal-assaultive group, found that the suicidal group were more likely to have a history of physical and, to a lesser degree, sexual abuse. Pfeffer *et al.* suggest that in treating suicidal adolescents it is important to consider the possibility of previous abuse, and to either intervene in the family to ensure the abuse does not continue or to remove the adolescent from the environment where the abuse has occurred. Clearly, neither option is simple.

Substance abuse and suicidal behaviour

We have already discussed that adolescents who exhibit suicide behaviour are likely to have few friends (Curran 1987). Some adolescents who find themselves isolated from their peers turn to mood-enhancing substances as a way of belonging. Parry-Jones (1985) describes the typical solvent abuser as 'lonely and friendless', and Pallikkathayil and Tweed (1983) suggest that many drug abusers use drugs as a means of being able to identify with a peer group (see Chapter 8 for a full account). The relationship between these two variables in relation to suicidal behaviour remains confounded but both have been implicated as being predictive of potential suicide behaviour in adolescents. Mussen *et al.* (1990) suggest that adolescents who abuse drugs or alcohol are more likely to engage in suicide behaviour and Pfeffer *et al.* (1989) found that adolescents who were suicidal, but not suicidal and assaultive, were more likely to have a history of substance or alcohol misuse.

There are however two quite separate groups of adolescents who attempt suicide whilst misusing drugs and alcohol. The first group are those with previous psychiatric disturbance who misuse substances as a means of maladaptive coping. These young people are more likely to make planned (and very serious) attempts at suicide (Shaffer 1985). They are frequently successful in their attempts. The second group are adolescents who misuse substances in response to an isolated event and, in a state of altered mood, will attempt suicide. Whilst these adolescents are less likely to be successful in their attempts, and typically choose less lethal methods, their attempts should nevertheless be taken seriously, and steps taken to resolve the precipitating crisis.

A further group of adolescents who typically abuse drugs are anorectics and bulimics who misuse substances as a way of purging. Suicide behaviour among this group is also high. Viesselman and Roig (1985) found that nearly 40% of their sample of anorectics and bulimics had made past suicidal gestures. A study by Woolf and Gren (1990), which looked at acute poisoning among female adolescent anorectics, showed them to be a worrying group because, typically, they delay in seeking help after overdose of substances.

School factors

The importance and influence of school in the lives of adolescents cannot be underestimated. Not only do adolescents spend a good deal of time at school, they are also likely to derive their friends and peers from within the school population.

Parents, particularly those from higher socioeconomic groups, tend to place great emphasis upon academic success and upon popularity at school (Conger 1991). Failure at school therefore can leave the adolescent with a sense of having 'let parents down', and changing school can remove from the adolescent the important buffer of friends and peers, leading to a feeling of isolation and loneliness. Both factors appear to have some significance in the study of suicide behaviour.

It is however, very difficult to separate school factors from the wider social context within which the adolescent functions. School failure, for example, may lead to parental conflict and pressure by parents to succeed can result in high levels of anxiety, and subsequent failure. What is apparent in studies of suicide behaviour is that school failure is an important factor in suicide behaviour (Adams and Adams 1991; Conger 1991). Failure should be monitored carefully and handled sensitively, particularly if parental expectations are high. Additionally, Mussen *et al.* (1990) suggest that a declining school performance can also be indicative of potential suicide behaviour. As well as failing in terms of academic achievement, being caught in delinquent or antisocial acts (such as truancy) has also been associated with potential suicide behaviour. Schaffer (1974), in a study of inquest records of 30 suicides in children aged between 7 and 15 years, found that one of the most commonly referred to precipitating factors was fear of parents finding out about delinquent behaviour at school.

The final factor implicated in studies relating to adolescent suicide is changing school. We have already discussed throughout this book the importance of friends, and it is difficult to ascertain whether changing school is a significant factor, or if it further represents the importance of losing friends and peers. However, both Pfeffer *et al.* (1989) and Adams and Adams (1991) found that going to a new school is associated with suicide behaviour, which suggests that adolescents are vulnerable at this time. These studies have particular importance in relation to adolescents who have to change schools frequently due, for example, to parental occupation. Further research in this area is clearly warranted.

Prevention of suicide behaviour in adolescents

The discussion in the previous section has highlighted those warning signs which may be significant in suicide behaviour during adolescence. It is by no means a complete discussion, however, nor could it ever be. There will always be adolescents (and adults) who take, or attempt to take their own lives, who will not exhibit warning signs or fit into high risk classifications. The problem is perhaps confounded by the fact that most suicide prevention strategies require an element of self-referral, and serious suicide attempters will clearly be reluctant to seek help which may prevent them from ending their own lives.

As discussed in the previous section, however, there has been a great deal of work undertaken which has identified warning signs in relation to adolescent suicide behaviour and which can be utilized to identify those adolescents who are most at risk. Specific intervention can then be directed to those who most need help. Reducing the rate of suicide has been placed high on the agenda by the Department of Health in their document *The Health of the Nation* (DoH 1992).

Nurses working in schools, teachers and general practitioners are in ideal positions to detect young people who appear depressed, or who are potentially at risk because of, for example, their family circumstances. There are however more structured ways of identifying young people at risk, and preventative models from the United States, Canada and Sweden provide useful data on how preventative programmes could be utilized.

School prevention programmes

Over the last decade in the United States and Canada, as the number of adolescent suicides has increased, various school-based prevention programmes have been set up (Reynolds 1991; Lamb and Pusker 1991; see also Tierney *et al.* 1990). These programmes have attempted to use psychometric assessment scales to measure risk. Setting up such a programme is complex and not all have been able to demonstrate true efficacy (Reynolds 1991). However, by combining psychometric assessment scales with follow-up interviews, identification of at-risk adolescents is feasible (Lamb and Pusker 1991; Reynolds 1991; Beer and Beer 1992). Examples of scales used are the *Suicide Ideation Questionnaire* and the *Adolescent Depression Scale* (see Reynolds 1991), and the *Self-Analysis Questionnaire* designed by Spielberger (see Lamb and Pusker 1991). Reynolds (1991) suggests that adolescents identified as being at risk should be further screened and suggests the use of the *Suicide Behaviors Interview (SBI)* which is a semi-structured clinical interview which allows the gathering of data relating to specific problems and stressors, and can subsequently direct the nature of referral or support. The SBI has been shown to have high reliability and internal validity and it is somewhat disappointing that wider trials using this and other techniques have not been undertaken.

Identification of at-risk adolescents, however, is only the first stage towards prevention. Tierney *et al* (1990) suggest that programmes must consist of prevention, intervention and postvention. *Prevention* of suicide involves enhancing problem solving and coping skills which, according to Tierney *et al.* (1990), can be undertaken as part of the school curriculum. There are many opportunities for encouraging the development of such skills, in a variety of subject areas. *Intervention* involves the early identification of suicide potential among individual students, and referring at-risk young people to appropriate agencies. *Postvention* refers to the process by which adolescents are helped to cope after a suicide has occurred in the school.

Instigating a school-based prevention programme is, as we have already mentioned, complex. If such programmes are to effective, they involve planning and resourcing. It should not be assumed, for example, that teachers and nurses possess the necessary skills for the identification of adolescents at risk, or for coping with these young people after they have been identified (Duffy 1993). They will require specific training which will inevitably be costly in terms of both time and money. We would suggest, however, that if the governments target for a reduction in suicide is to be achieved then some investment is inevitable. There is also a potential role for community psychiatric nurses in schools who could, according to Lamb and Pusker (1991) open 'new avenues to the promotion of adolescent mental health' (p103). Furthermore, Tierney *et al.* (1990) suggest that it is not only teachers and nurses who require specific training but any one who is in contact with students in the school environment including secretarial staff, cafeteria staff and bus drivers, as well as parents. They also stress the importance of a school climate which promotes openness and trust between adolescents and staff, which is a clear prerequisite to a successful programme.

A further essential component of a successful school-based prevention programme is the prompt referral of at risk adolescents to agencies which are able to provide support and counselling. This involves close and formal liaison with, for example, community mental health services (Tierney *et al.* 1990; Lamb and Pusker 1991). Hodgman and McAnarney (1992) suggest that, where an adolescent shows signs of serious suicide intent, hospitalization is essential, so that prompt and continuous support can be offered.

Our final point in relation to school-based programmes relates to intervention in the unfortunate event of a suicide among the school population, and possibly in relation to highly publicized suicide by people outside the school. The importance of this point was highlighted in a study in the United States by Phillips and Carstensen (cited in Buskist and Gerbing 1990) who studied the relationship between 38 nationally televized suicides or feature stories of adolescent suicide and the incidence of adolescent suicide during the following week. The study which was carried out over a six year period found a significant rise in suicide rates among adolescents, suggesting that media focus on suicide can precipitate suicide behaviour among young people. The immediate management of the suicide is then clearly important, and in the case of suicide among school colleagues involves making decisions about, for example, how and when students will be told about the death of one of their peers and funeral arrangements. Providing individual and group counselling so that adolescents can vent their feeling is also clearly an important strategic intervention (Tierney *et al.* 1990). In view of the government's wish to reduce suicide we would therefore suggest that serious thought be given to the development of school-based prevention programmes. It is interesting to note that in some parts of the United States such programmes are required by law (see Tierney *et al.* 1990) and, whilst they may be expensive to develop, the investment is small compared with the devastation of an unnecessary and preventable death of a young person. Furthermore, there is no evidence to suggest that suicide prevention programmes are in any way harmful. Screening for suicide behaviour does not appear to carry any risk of increased suicide behaviour (Hodgman and McAnarney 1992).

Suicide prevention in general practice

Apart from nurses and others who have contact with young people in schools, those involved in general practice are also ideally situated to detect suicide risk among adolescents. Hodgman and McAnarney (1992) suggest however that symptoms of depression and suicidality in adolescent patients are frequently overlooked, particularly by doctors in general practice. There is clearly a need to improve assessment in primary practice and nurses who work in this sphere should, as well as doctors, be aware that the young people they come into contact with may be at risk. Early research by Barraclough *et al.* (1974) suggests that the majority of people who commit suicide seek consultation with their doctors in the period preceding their deaths. There is no evidence to suggest that the situation today is any different.

As we have suggested in relation to school-based personnel there is clear evidence to support suicide awareness training among those involved in general practice. A study in Sweden (Rutz *et al.* 1989), which measured the effect of a suicide awareness programme directed at general practitioners, showed positive results. Michel and Valach (1992) also demonstrated that training programmes in suicide prevention made a significant difference to the attitudes and knowledge of general practitioners.

In view of the enhanced role of practice nurses, we would suggest that such programmes should be made available to them also because they come into contact with patients as part of their practice. Practice nurses may also be able to participate in screening programmes for adolescents which have been shown to be useful in identifying problems among adolescents in general practice (Donovan and McCarthy 1988).

Caring for parasuicidal adolescents

In relation to this discussion of adolescent suicide, we feel it is important to discuss the care of those who have attempted suicide and have subsequently come into contact with the health services. There is little empirical evidence which gives guidance into the effective management of adolescents who exhibit suicide behaviour. Indeed, a great deal of research into the management of both adolescent and adult parasuicide is highly critical of the care they receive. In an audit of accident and emergency services in Leicester for adolescent parasuicide patients, O'Dwyer *et al.* (1991) found that care was generally unsatisfactory, with almost a third of the subjects studied being discharged from the accident and emergency facility with no psychiatric consultation or follow-up. Only 51% were admitted to hospital. As a result of this study, accident and emergency doctors in Leicester are now actively encouraged to seek the advice of the child psychiatry services. However, other data suggest that the care of parasuicide patients in accident and emergency departments remains unsatisfactory. Dunleavey (1992), Palmer (1993) and Lindars (1991) found that care tended to focus on physical needs and nurses appeared unable (or unwilling) to provide psychological or social support. Lindars (1991) found that this was particularly so when drug abusers were admitted after taking overdoses.

The care of parasuicide patients admitted to general hospital wards was also found to be lacking. In a study of parasuicide patients in a London hospital, Dunleavey (1992) found that nurses tended to isolate these patients and deny them human contact. One patient in this study remarked that the staff 'just sort of saved you and put you in a corner' (p214). Dunleavey suggests that isolation and castigation was the norm and that hospital became an extension of the ordeal of parasuicide, rather than becoming a place where therapy could really commence.

Parasuicide patients clearly require care that is sensitive and which addresses the emotional trauma they are experiencing. Lindars (1991) suggests that all parasuicide patients should be given skilled psychiatric help, which could feasibly be provided by community psychiatric nurses. Evans *et al.* (1992) discuss one such exemplar of good practice which involves a parasuicide service at a London hospital. Specialist psychiatric nurses assess parasuicide patients and make decisions about the most suitable follow-up arrangements (i.e. psychiatric admission or outpatient follow-up). Patients who are discharged are given contact numbers in case of emergency. The service has been extremely successful during its five year period of existence. Such a service as that outlined by Evans *et al.* (1992) is obviously desirable and inexpensive when compared with the cost of in-patient admission and human suffering. Parasuicide patients will, however, still need to be cared for on either paediatric or general medicine wards and the care they receive must be of a high standard. When on the general ward, patients should be encouraged to mix with other people and isolation should be avoided. Nurses in ward areas, as well as in accident and emergency departments, should provide holistic care, which includes meeting the psychosocial needs of the individual (Palmer 1993). Nurses should, furthermore, be encouraged to explore their own attitudes towards parasuicide patients, and should be aware of the potential effects their attitudes may have on the quality of care they deliver.

Implications for nurses

The implications for nurses involved in the care of adolescents are many and the lack of British research into the area of adolescent suicide and suicide behaviour is worrying, particularly if the Department of Health's targets in relation to suicide are to be achieved by the end of the century. Areas of concern involve school nurses and community psychiatric nurses who should be striving to ensure that school-based suicide prevention programmes are set up. There are several examples of good practice in this area in the United States which we have mentioned in the preceding sections of this chapter. Practice nurses should also be aware of the need to assess their adolescent patients, who may appear at the surgery for seemingly insignificant reasons but who may be in severe psychological distress and at risk of suicide behaviour. Secondly, when prevention programmes fail and adolescents do attempt suicide, nurses in accident and emergency departments and in hospital wards should recognize that psychological therapy commences from the moment the young person enters the hospital. Parasuicide has replaced the term 'attempted suicide' because of the connotations of failure implicit in the terms 'attempted' (Palmer 1993). Young parasuicide patients are already likely to be lacking in self-esteem and may perceive their failure to have succeeded in suicide as yet another thing they were unable to achieve success with. The attitudes of nurses can do a great deal to help the distressed adolescent and sensitive, empathetic care is essential. Unfortunately much of the research we have reviewed shows that care is often judgemental and the psychosocial needs of the patient are frequently ignored. This situation remains puzzling to us, particularly in view of the great advances that have made in terms of holistic nursing care over the past decade. It may be that nurses feel in some ways threatened by parasuicide, or that caring for those who are considered to be 'psychiatric' patients in general hospitals, as highlighted by Stockwell (1972), remains problematic for nurses. Whatever the reasons we hope that more research will be undertaken which can highlight not only the special needs of this vulnerable group, but also the most effective ways in which nurses can provide care.

References

Adams, M. and Adams, J. (1991) Life events, depression and perceived problem solving alternatives in adolescents. *Journal of Child Psychology and Psychiatry*, 32(5): 811–820.

Barraclough, B., Bunch, J., Nelson, B. and Sainsbury, P. (1974) A hundred cases of suicide: clinical aspects. *British Journal of Psychiatry*, 125: 355–373.

Beer, J. and Beer, J. (1992) Depression, self-esteem, suicide ideation and GPAs of high school students at risk. *Psychological Reports*, 71(3): 899–902.

Briere, J., Evans, D., Runtz, M. and Wall, T. (1988) Symptomology in men who were abused as children: a comparison study. *American Journal of Orthopsychiatry*, 58: 457–461.

Buskist, W. and Gerbing, D.N. (1990) *Psychology: Boundaries and Frontiers.* Scott Foresman/Little, Brown, Illinois.

Conger, J.J. (1991) *Adolescence and Youth*, 4th edn. Harper Collins, New York.

Curran, D.K. (1987) *Adolescent Suicidal Behavior.* Hemisphere Publishing, Washington DC.

Department of Health (1992) *The Health of the Nation.* HMSO, London.

Deykin, E.Y., Alpert, J.J. and McNamarra, J.J. (1985) A pilot study of the effect of exposure to child abuse or neglect on adolescent suicidal behavior. *American Journal of Psychiatry*, 142: 1299–1303.

Donovan, C.F. and McCarthy, S. (1988) Is there a place for screening in general practice? *Health Trends*, 20: 64–65.

Duffy, D. (1993) Preventing suicide. *Nursing Times*, 89(31): 28–31.

Dunleavey, R. (1992) An adequate response to a cry for help: parasuicide patients' perceptions of their nursing care. *Professional Nurse*, 7(4): 213–215.

Durkheim, E. (1952 translation) *Suicide: A Study in Sociology.* Routledge and Kegan Paul, London.

Erikson, E. (1965) *Childhood and Society.* Penguin, Harmondsworth.

Evans, M., Cox, C. and Turnbull, G. (1992) Parasuicide response. *Nursing Times*, 88(19): 34–36.

Goodwin, J. (1981) Suicide attempts in sexual abuse victims and their mothers. *Child Abuse and Neglect*, 5: 217–221.

Grotevant, H.D. and Cooper, C.R. (1985) Patterns of interaction in family relationships and the development of identity exploration in adolescence. *Child Development*, 56: 415–428.

Gunn, S. (1987) Helping parents to cope with adolescents. *Health at School*, 3(3): 76–77.

Hartup, W.W. (1989) Social relationships and their significance. *American Psychologist*, 44: 120–126.

Hempel, S. (1992) Suicide: facts pack. *Community Outlook*, August: 16–17.

Hodgman, C.H. and McAnarney, E.R. (1992) Adolescent depression and suicide: rising problems. *Hospital Practice*, 27(4): 73–96.

Lamb, J. and Pusker, K.R. (1991) School-based adolescent mental health project survey of depression, suicidal ideation, and anger. *Journal of Child and Adolescent Psychiatric and Mental Health Nursing*, 4(3): 101–104.

Laufer, M. (1974) *Adolescent Disturbance and Breakdown.* Penguin Books in association with MIND, Harmondsworth.

Lindars, J. (1991) Holistic care in parasuicide. *Nursing Times*, 87(15): 30–31.

Lowenstein, I.F. (1990) Suicide and self-destructive behaviour in adolescents. *Health at School*, 5(5): 155–157.

Marcia, J.E. (1982) Identity in adolescence. In: *Handbook of Adolescent Psychology.* (Ed. J. Adelson) John Wiley, Chichester.

McClure, G.M. (1988) Suicide in children in England and Wales. *Journal of Child Psychology and Psychiatry*, 29(3): 345–349.

McCormack, A., Janus, M. and Burgess, A.W. (1986) Runaway youths and sexual victimisation: gender differences in an adolescent runaway population. *Child Abuse and Neglect*, 10: 387–395.

Michel, K. and Valach, L. (1992) Suicide prevention: spreading the gospel to general practitioners. *British Journal of Psychiatry*, 160: 757–760.

Mussen, P.H., Conger, J.J., Kagan, J. and Huston, A.C. (1990) *Child Development and Personality*, 7th edn. Harper and Row, New York.

Myers, K., McCauley, E., Calderon, R. and Treder, R. (1991) The 3-year longitudinal course of suicidality and predictive factors for subsequent suicidality in youths with major depressive disorder. *Journal of the American Academy of Child Psychiatry*, 30: 804–810.

O'Dwyer, F.G., D'Alton, A. and Pearce, J.B. (1991) Adolescent self harm patients: audit of assessment in an accident and emergency department. *British Medical Journal*, 303: 629–630.

OPCS (1983–1993) *Mortality Statistics: Cause. England and Wales Series Nos. DH2 Nos. 8–19*. HMSO, London.

Pallikkathayil, L. and Tweed, S. (1983) Substance abuse: alcohol and drugs during adolescence. *The Nursing Clinics of North America*, 18(2): 313–321.

Palmer, S. (1993) Para-suicide: a cause for nursing concern. *Nursing Standard*, 7(19): 37–39.

Parry-Jones, W.L1. Adolescent disturbance. In: *Child and Adolescent Psychiatry*, 2nd edn. (Eds M. Rutter and L. Hersov) Blackwell Scientific Publications, Oxford.

Pfeffer, C.R., Newcorn, J., Kaplan, G., Mizruchi, M.S. and Plutchik, R. (1989) Subtypes of suicide and assaultive behaviors in adolescent psychiatric inpatients: a research note. *Journal of Child Psychology and Psychiatry*, 30(1): 151–163.

Reynolds, W.M. (1989) *Reynolds Adolescent Depression Scale (RADS): Professional Manual*. Psychological Assessment Resources, Odessa, Florida.

Reynolds, W.M. (1991) A school-based procedure for the identification of adolescents at risk for suicidal behaviour. *Family and Community Health*, 14(3): 64–75.

Rutz, W., van Knorning, L. and Walinder, L. (1989) Frequency of suicide on Gotland after systematic post-graduate education of general practitioners. *Acta Psychiatrica Scandinavica*, 80: 151–154.

Seligman, M.E.P. and Peterson, C. (1986) A learned helplessness perspective on childhood depression: theory and research. In: *Depression in Young People: Developmental and Clinical Perspectives*. (Eds M. Rutter, C. Izard and P. Read) Guilford Press, New York.

Selman, R.L. (1981) The child as a friendship philosopher. In: *The Development of Children's Friendships*. (Eds S.R. Asher and J.M.Cottman) Cambridge University Press, New York.

Shaffer, D. (1974) Suicide in childhood and early adolescence. *Journal of Child Psychology and Psychiatry*, 15: 275–291.

Shaffer, D. (1985) Depression, mania and suicidal acts. In: *Child and Adolescent Psychiatry*, 2nd edn. (Eds M. Rutter and L. Hersov) Blackwell Scientific Publications, Oxford.

Singer, K.I. (1989) Group work with men who experienced incest in childhood. *American Journal of Orthopsychiatry*, 59: 468–472.

Steinberg, D. (1987) *Basic Adolescent Psychiatry*. Blackwell Scientific Publications, Oxford.

Stockwell, F. (1972) *The Unpopular Patient*. RCN, London.

Tierney, R., Ramsay, R., Tanney, B. and Lang, W. (1990) Comprehensive school suicide prevention programmes. *Death Studies*, 14(4): 347–370.

Viesselman, J.O. and Roig, M. (1985) Depression and suicidality in eating disorders. *Journal of Clinical Psychiatry*, 46: 118–124.

Walker, M., Moreau, D. and Weissman, M.M. (1990) Parents' awareness of children's suicide attempts. *American Journal of Psychiatry*, 147: 1364–1366.

Watkins, B. and Bentovim, A. (1992) The sexual abuse of male children and adolescents: a review of current research. *Journal of Child Psychology and Psychiatry*, 33(1): 197–248.

Woolf, A.D. and Gren, J.M. (1990) Acute poisonings among adolescents and young adults with anorexia nervosa. *American Journal of Diseases of Children*, 144(7): 785–788.

World Health Organization (1990) *World Health Statistical Annual*. WHO, Geneva.

Youniss, J. and Smollar, J. (1985) *Adolescent Relations with Mothers, Fathers and Friends*. University of Chicago Press, Chicago.

Further reading

Conrad, N. (1991) Where do they turn? *Journal of Psychosocial Nursing*, 29(3): 14–20.

A useful article which highlights some of the epidemiological data from the USA. Conrad investigates family, health and religious variables in relation to suicide ideation.

Pfeffer, C.R. (1986) *The Suicidal Child*. Guilford Press, New York.

A stimulating book which is easy to read and which covers the subject of child suicide in a thorough and sensitive way.

Tierney, R., Ramsay, R., Tanney, B. and Lang, W. (1990) Comprehensive school suicide prevention programmes. *Death Studies*, 14(4): 347–370.

This article addresses responses to suicide by school systems in North America, and discusses school-based prevention programmes. It is useful reading for school nurses and teachers who are concerned about the issue of adolescent suicide.

Chapter 11
The Challenge for Researchers

It is inevitable that at the end of a book of this kind the authors make a plea for there to be more research into the field under consideration. There are so many outstanding questions unanswered that this book is no exception. The difference is perhaps that at the present time the opportunities to formulate research projects in the field of providing health care and nursing for adolescents are enormous. Rarely has such a broad specialism within nursing received so little serious attention from researchers not only in the UK but to some extent worldwide.

During the last decade nurses have become supportive of the need for research and through major initiatives in upgrading their basis for training, have committed themselves to reviewing and implementing where possible the results of research findings. There is now a much greater awareness of the significance of research to the professional standing of the nursing profession. This supportive approach to research has enabled a wider commitment to providing underpinning knowledge to enhance clinical practice. Yet even within this supportive environment there are few well known researchers working in the field of the provision of nursing care to adolescents. This is further evidence of the need to bring together committed individuals to research this important field.

It may be that we should be advocating for a separate speciality akin to psychiatrists who specialize in adolescent mental health issues. There is no doubt however that the nursing care needs of adolescents are of prime relevance to all four branches of nursing and to midwifery. This alone warrants much further consideration of the needs of adolescents both in terms of promoting healthy lifestyles and in the provision of appropriate health care.

What needs to be done?

It is relatively easy to identify broad fields for further research but more difficult to prioritize major issues which need further detailed consideration. This in fact might be a useful piece of empirical work to carry out anyway to help establish what it is we need to do next in order to improve the provision of nursing care for adolescents. Our list reflects our own interests and biases but also we hope does overlap to some extent with yours.

The health needs of adolescence

We believe that it remains of major importance to further clarify the nature of adolescence. Chapters 1 and 2 highlight the difficulties in providing nursing care to a group which is difficult to determine other than through quasi-legal definitions. The important issue to us is to try and understand better how adolescents see themselves and their perspective on how best to provide nursing care. Individuals tend to know how they fit more comfortably into externally created situations which is clearly the case when adolescents are hospitalized.

There is a further issue here which reflects the broadness of the use of the term 'adolescence'. As the reader will know most textbooks on developmental psychology include considerable information on childhood during which so many physiological and cognitive changes occur, but adolescence and ageing are often covered in one or at the most two chapters. It seems to us that there is a case for developing more sophisticated approaches to the study of adolescence which reflect the increasing amount of literature in this field. There seems to us a major difference between those adolescents emerging from childhood and experiencing being a teenager and those young adults with adolescent leanings who are often in further or higher education or starting work.

To some, adolescence can spread through until such time as a major life event initiates change, such as the birth of the first child or the death of a parent or guardian. Clearly, this is in part mediated by individual differences (Chapter 3) but nevertheless seems to reflect better the knowledge and research findings this text has brought together. We strongly advocate a more sophisticated analysis of the notion of adolescence as seen through the eyes of adolescents themselves. This may provide further information to help nurses provide the most effective forms of health care for the wide range of young people encompassed by the broad category covering adolescence.

Health promotion in adolescents

Adolescence remains a time for learning and experimenting. Young people want to try and find out exactly what it is to be adult and often sample a number of adult activities. These include smoking and drinking alcohol as well as more risky behaviours as described in Chapters 8 and 9. The serious consequences of these behaviours are well documented and indeed are likely to be familiar to young people. What is more difficult is developing intervention strategies to effectively change behaviour. It is clear that we need to develop health promotion strategies which utilize the knowledge and experience adolescents already have and to evaluate their effectiveness. Furthermore, we need to create environments which make certain behaviours acceptable within clear constraints. Adolescents are building up their own value system and need to be encouraged to explore options within limits whilst coming to terms with the fact that certain behaviours are unhealthy and indeed dangerous.

There is the need to concentrate future research on the effectiveness of different approaches to intervention and to develop a specialist field in adolescent health promotion. This is likely to be interdisciplinary and to draw upon the skills and expertise of a wide range of professionals including nurses, youth workers and teachers. Legislation alone is unlikely to be the most effective approach nor can we expect persuasion from barely credible adults to make a great impact. Instead we need to research and explore new approaches which start from how young people perceive health and which embrace them in the process as sophisticated field researchers. This is a real challenge to some of the more conventional approaches towards health promotion but one which is likely to set more realistic goals for health promotion.

Impact of illness on young adults

This is clearly a very important topic to research and understand more clearly. All of us experience ill health in different ways and develop our own strategies with which to cope with such difficulties. To some adolescents experiencing chronic illness, this adjustment is long rather than short term. This book has brought together research findings and studies in the field of adolescent behaviour. This forms a useful base from which to study individual reactions and perhaps more importantly to develop methodologies which help determine them in the clinical environments. There are numerous studies which investigate the needs of younger people both prior and during hospitalization. There is a strong and well developed body of knowledge which has demonstrated the importance of preparing young children for hospitalization and indeed for creating the right environment in which to facilitate their health care. There are few, if any, such studies with adolescents, which reflects the paucity of research in this field and perhaps the difficulty in defining adolescent behaviour. If, to some extent, we are prepared to allow adolescents themselves to determine their own level of maturity and health needs this would provide a stronger framework within which to provide different forms of health care for this client group.

Evaluating different health care options

It is clear that there is not one approach which suits all individuals when facing ill health. There are therefore a variety of approaches to providing health care most of which however relate primarily to children or adults. The options which would appear to be available for young people tend to have been derived from administrative convenience rather than a careful assessment and evaluation of the needs of the adolescent group. Hence, as discussed earlier in this book in some situations adolescents might find themselves being cared for with children and in other situations being placed on adult wards. Nor are there many specialized services set up to provide direct support for adolescence. In recognizing this it is important to try and develop innovative approaches to providing health care. This might be through offering specialized wards for adolescents which despite the additional costs in establishing such provision might indeed be a more economic option in the long term if it improves health care. Other approaches might be to focus much more on community provision and perhaps through engaging other external agencies such as education and social services to provide a more comprehensive support service which is more readily in line with adolescent behaviour. There are other alternatives which need reviewing.

It is recognized that providing services of this kind cannot be without cost. Furthermore, given the current situation within the agencies providing health care it is extremely difficult to set up new provision of this kind which has not been evaluated and indeed might be very costly. And yet unless initiatives relating to the provision of alternative approaches to health are developed the current level of services will continue rather than evolve. We would like to encourage service managers and budget holders to take seriously the needs of the adolescent client group in the context of the changing health care needs of the nation, and to recognize that time and resources invested in this group might well be for the long term benefit not only for the individuals themselves but to the effect of running health services.

The long term effects on families

There has been extensive research into the effects of individual illness on families. This has highlighted, particularly in the fields of adult ill health, the difficulties experienced by family members often as carers as well as indirectly by being part of the family. Hence, for example, victims of head injury or stroke often impact greatly upon the family dynamics. This has led to the view that any illness or impairment that directly affects one family member impacts greatly upon others. The 'patient' in a medical sense is not only the individual with ill health but the extended family network which is directly affected.

The research in this field is indeed sparse. And yet the impact which adolescent illness has on family networks may be enormous. It is inevitable that parents and carers or guardians have an immediate responsibility for supporting the young person throughout the illness. At the same time this may impact greatly on their own lives and indeed the lives of elderly relatives for whom they may be providing care and their peers. The changes which adolescent illness bring about to the normal pattern of family life can in some cases be traumatic. Even for the most minor of illnesses the changes to the family can be great and the psychological impact enormous. There are always concerns which parents feel the most when young people are unwell especially when hospitalized or receiving health care other than through a general practitioner.

In some cases the impact is over an extended period of time. This will involve changes in lifestyles both for the parents or guardians and all those who are part of the family network. In a severe case it may mean changes in occupation or short term changes in lifestyle, which might have long term influences on the family economic position. Changes such as these cannot be under estimated and it is not unlikely that the way in which a family copes with adolescent illness influences the ways in which the adults themselves are able to adjust. This area of research is much neglected and it is now opportune to prioritize work in this field at a time when greater emphasis is being placed upon the provision of community care.

Approaching research

More than ever there is now a strong case for research into the provision of health care to be carried out on an interdisciplinary basis. Central to the interdisciplinary team is the expertise and knowledge which the nurse can bring. The changing patterns of initial nurse training and in service education opportunities have equipped us with a well qualified and committed nursing personnel. It is now important to utilize these skills in enhancing the provision of nursing care. The range of opportunities and approaches are relatively well defined and provide an important basis from which to contribute more widely to this field of work.

Case studies

The collecting of careful case study material, whether descriptively or on an experimental basis, is one means of bringing together important research data. Many nurses are well placed to carry out work of this kind. Carefully planned and objectively analysed case studies are an invaluable source of material, both for the development of a broader knowledge base and for the planning of future health care provision. Series of descriptive or experimental case studies can be brought together into a more coherent framework within which broader generalizations can be drawn. Research of this kind has been much neglected and, in applied health care settings, can be a rich and easily accessible means of informing practice.

Longitudinal studies

Case studies as described above can lead to longitudinal research. However, more often than not it is essential to bring together a more comprehensive and detailed framework within which to carry out longitudinal work. The value of longitudinal studies is that they enable changing patterns of behaviour to be plotted and to enable a rapport to be built up with the research sample. In some ways the ability to carry out longitudinal studies often depends on gaining external funding. It is possible nevertheless within nursing areas where long term care is being provided to develop small but nevertheless important studies. Individual change over a period of time is an important influence on the provision of health care and as has been pointed out already the period of adolescence is one of considerable change.

Cross sectional studies

Cross sectional studies enable comparisons between different groups to be made without the need for carrying out longitudinal research. It would be possible on this basis to sample a group of young adolescents at onset of a particular illness; during hospitalization at an agreed point; and at some period after discharge. Studies of this kind are more common in the research literature and are indeed easier to carry out than longitudinal work. They are in fact cheaper and quicker to complete as it is not necessary to have the same sample for each part of the data collection. Providing sample characteristics are similar, broad generalizations can be drawn. The value of studies of this kind are not insignificant and certainly in the broader fields of behaviourial sciences, especially psychology, have been very influential in building up a strong body of knowledge. Supported by case studies and where longitudinal research may be possible, this approach provides a very powerful tool for nursing professions.

Applied evaluative research

Although not a specific research methodology the need to carry out evaluative research and techniques required is becoming of major importance to policy makers and the providers of health care. Evaluation research focuses on a range of variables including making judgements about different kinds of health care provision; matching individuals to different approaches in the provision of nursing care; comparing different approaches both in the short term and the long term and in many cases collecting data on the efficiency of different approaches, often through analysis of cost options. There is the need within this area of work for nurses themselves to develop the skills of evaluation research and to set their expertise within this broader perspective.

Action research

Characteristic of the approaches outlined above is fostering the professional commitment in nurses carrying out research. Research is an important aspect of the role of all professionals engaged in the provision of services. Nurses as action researchers, where their skills on a day-to-day basis are structured in such a way as to enable empirical information to be brought together to influence future practice, are a critical component of the further professionalization of nursing. Historically nursing research has often been carried out by other professionals including those from the biological and behaviourial sciences. The emerging research trend is for interdisciplinary research with the prime focus on data collection being within the ownership of the nurse practitioner. This is almost the strongest model with which to provide good information on which to base future health care judgements in the care of the adolescent.

Conclusion

This text has brought together a wide range of work in the field of adolescence. It has been written from an interdisciplinary perspective bringing together the background and experience of the authors in the fields of nursing, child and adolescent behaviour, and the psychological sciences. It is aimed at encouraging those who are providing health care to adolescents to develop a stronger research base from which to make professional judgements. The authors themselves believe this area of work is much defected and are concerned that historical neglect might lead to a lowering of the priority given to supporting this particular group. It is believed that, by empowering the nursing profession and through encouraging a wider dissemination of the needs of adolescents, this will be avoided. The most effective way of doing this is without doubt to encourage development of research and to provide data and information pertinent to the needs of decision making processes of policy makers. It is hoped that the reader, whatever his or her speciality, will recognize the importance of providing health care to adolescents and through their own professional practice would encourage and stimulate research into this important field.

Further reading

Dixon, G. *et al.* (1995) Disability in late adolescence III: Utilisation of health services. *Disability and Rehabilitation*, in Press.

Hirst, M. and Baldwin, S. (1994) *Unequal Opportunities. Growing up Disabled.* HMSO, London.

Langley, J.D. *et al.* (1995) Disability in late adolescence I: Introduction, methods and overview. *Disability and Rehabilitation*, in Press.

Stanton, W.R., Langley, J. and McGee, R. (1995) Disability in late adolescence II: Follow-up of perceived limitation. *Disability and Rehabilitation*, in Press.

Appendix
Useful Addresses

Advice, Advocacy and Representation Service for Children
1 Sickle Street, Manchester   M60 2AA.

AL-ANON
61 Great Dover Street, London   SE1 4YS.

Anti-Bullying Campaign
10 Borough High Street, London   SE1 9QQ.

Brook Advisory Centre
153A East Street, London   SE17 2SD.

Childline
Royal Mail Building, Studd Street, London   N1 0QW.

Disabled Living Foundation
380–384 Harrow Road, London   W9 2HU.

Eating Disorders Association
Sackville Place, 44 Magdalen Street, Norwich   NR3 1JU.

Narcotics Anonymous
P.O. Box 1980, London   N19 3LS.

National Council of YMCAs
640 Forest Road, London   E17 3DZ.

RE-SOLV
30A High Street, Stone, Staffordshire   ST15 8AW

Index